MENTAL HEALTH, SUBSTANCE USE, and WELLBEING in HIGHER EDUCATION

Supporting the Whole Student

Alan I. Leshner and Layne A. Scherer, *Editors*

Committee on Mental Health, Substance Use, and Wellbeing
in STEMM Undergraduate and Graduate Education

Board on Higher Education and Workforce
Policy and Global Affairs

Board on Health Sciences Policy
Health and Medicine Division

A Consensus Study Report of

The National Academies of
SCIENCES · ENGINEERING · MEDICINE

THE NATIONAL ACADEMIES PRESS
Washington, DC
www.nap.edu

THE NATIONAL ACADEMIES PRESS   500 Fifth Street, NW   Washington, DC 20001

This activity was supported by contracts between the National Academy of Sciences and the Substance Abuse and Mental Health Services Administration (SAMHSA) under award HHSP2333201400020B, the National Institute on Mental Health (NIMH), the National Institute on Drug Abuse (NIDA), and the National Institute on Alcohol Abuse and Alcoholism (NIAAA) under award HHSN263201800029I. Any opinions, findings, conclusions, or recommendations expressed in this publication do not necessarily reflect the views of any organization or agency that provided support for the project.

International Standard Book Number-13: 978-0-309-12412-6
International Standard Book Number-10: 0-309-12412-3
Digital Object Identifier: https://doi.org/10.17226/26015
Library of Congress Control Number: 2021930903

Additional copies of this publication are available from the National Academies Press, 500 Fifth Street, NW, Keck 360, Washington, DC 20001; (800) 624-6242 or (202) 334-3313; http://www.nap.edu.

Printed in the United States of America

Suggested citation: National Academies of Sciences, Engineering, and Medicine. 2021. *Mental Health, Substance Use, and Wellbeing in Higher Education: Supporting the Whole Student.* Washington, DC: The National Academies Press. https://doi.org/10.17226/26015.

The National Academies of
SCIENCES · ENGINEERING · MEDICINE

The **National Academy of Sciences** was established in 1863 by an Act of Congress, signed by President Lincoln, as a private, nongovernmental institution to advise the nation on issues related to science and technology. Members are elected by their peers for outstanding contributions to research. Dr. Marcia McNutt is president.

The **National Academy of Engineering** was established in 1964 under the charter of the National Academy of Sciences to bring the practices of engineering to advising the nation. Members are elected by their peers for extraordinary contributions to engineering. Dr. John L. Anderson is president.

The **National Academy of Medicine** (formerly the Institute of Medicine) was established in 1970 under the charter of the National Academy of Sciences to advise the nation on medical and health issues. Members are elected by their peers for distinguished contributions to medicine and health. Dr. Victor J. Dzau is president.

The three Academies work together as the **National Academies of Sciences, Engineering, and Medicine** to provide independent, objective analysis and advice to the nation and conduct other activities to solve complex problems and inform public policy decisions. The National Academies also encourage education and research, recognize outstanding contributions to knowledge, and increase public understanding in matters of science, engineering, and medicine.

Learn more about the National Academies of Sciences, Engineering, and Medicine at **www.nationalacademies.org**.

The National Academies of
SCIENCES · ENGINEERING · MEDICINE

Consensus Study Reports published by the National Academies of Sciences, Engineering, and Medicine document the evidence-based consensus on the study's statement of task by an authoring committee of experts. Reports typically include findings, conclusions, and recommendations based on information gathered by the committee and the committee's deliberations. Each report has been subjected to a rigorous and independent peer-review process and it represents the position of the National Academies on the statement of task.

Proceedings published by the National Academies of Sciences, Engineering, and Medicine chronicle the presentations and discussions at a workshop, symposium, or other event convened by the National Academies. The statements and opinions contained in proceedings are those of the participants and are not endorsed by other participants, the planning committee, or the National Academies.

For information about other products and activities of the National Academies, please visit www.nationalacademies.org/about/whatwedo.

Study Staff

LAYNE A. SCHERER, Study Director
MARILYN BAKER, Acting Study Director (September–December 2020)
JOHN VERAS, Senior Program Assistant
AUSTEN APPLEGATE, Research Associate
MIRIAM AKEJU, Christine Mirzayan Science and Technology Policy Fellow, 2020
ADRIANA COUREMBIS, Senior Financial Business Partner (until April 2020)
CLARA SAVAGE, Senior Financial Business Partner
BARDIA MASSOUDKHAN, Senior Financial Business Partner

Consultants

JOSEPH ALPER, Consultant writer
JENNIFER SAUNDERS, Consultant writer

Preface

The ability of students to succeed in higher education and beyond is dependent on their physical and mental wellbeing, and the nation's institutions of higher education are seeing increasing levels of mental illness, substance use, and other forms of emotional distress among their students. Some of the problematic trends have been ongoing for decades. Some have been exacerbated by the COVID-19 pandemic and resulting economic consequences. Some are the result of long-festering systemic racism in almost every sphere of American life that are becoming more widely acknowledged throughout society and must, at last, be addressed.

Although the causal factors for each have their own idiosyncratic solutions, the increase in mental health and related problems has put tremendous pressure on the capacity of existing traditional college counseling and other support systems to handle the need for their services, leading to what some have called a "mental health crisis" on college campuses. Whether this constitutes a genuine crisis or not may be debated, but there is no question that new approaches and strategies are needed to deal with the increasing demand for help. This report lays out a variety of possible strategies and approaches, based on the available evidence on the nature of the issues and what works in various situations.

Although the report includes an array of recommendations, no real progress will be made unless individual institutions decide to promote a climate that clearly values the wellbeing of every student. The overall tone for that campus-wide atmosphere must, of course, be articulated by the leadership—the president, the board of trustees, faculty leaders—but must also involve all sectors of the institution—faculty, staff, and students. Each has a role to play.

A part of that culture change will require devoting more resources to promoting mental wellbeing, and that need is coming at a terrible time. Financial resources at almost every institution are severely constrained. However, this issue is of sufficient importance that, if necessary, priorities should be reevaluated and rearranged. The impacts of this problem are critical and broad enough that ensuring the wellbeing of all students must be near the top of the priority list. Hopefully, this report will help articulate the need for additional resources and provide a basis for moving forward on this issue.

I am extremely grateful to my superb colleagues on the National Academies of Sciences, Engineering, and Medicine's committee that authored this report. Leading such an expert and committed group of scholars has been an extremely rewarding experience. I also want to express, on behalf of the whole committee, our gratitude to the exceptionally competent and dedicated staff of the National Academies and the many others cited in the acknowledgments that follow.

Alan I. Leshner (NAM), *Chair*
Committee on Mental Health, Substance Use, and Wellbeing
in STEMM Undergraduate and Graduate Education

Acknowledgments

The committee would like to thank the following staff members for their hard work and dedication in bringing this report to fruition: Layne Scherer, Austen Applegate, Marilyn Baker, Ashley Bear, and John Veras, as well as consultants Joseph Alper and Jennifer Saunders. Without their commitment, this report would not have been possible. The committee also thanks senior librarians Anne Marie Houppert and Rebecca Morgan, as well as the National Academies' research library, for assistance with fact checking and literature searches.

This Consensus Study Report was reviewed in draft form by individuals chosen for their diverse perspectives and technical expertise. The purpose of this independent review is to provide candid and critical comments that will assist the National Academies of Sciences, Engineering, and Medicine in making each published report as sound as possible and to ensure that it meets the institutional standards for quality, objectivity, evidence, and responsiveness to the study charge. The review comments and draft manuscript remain confidential to protect the integrity of the deliberative process.

We thank the following individuals for their review of this report: Amelia Arria, University of Maryland; Stephen Beckley, Hodgkins Beckley Consulting; Traci Callandrillo, American University; Kafui Dzirasa, Duke University; Patricia Frazier, University of Minnesota; Sylvia Gonzalez, Austin Community College; Renée Jenkins, Howard University; Julia Kent, Council of Graduate Schools; Emily Lattie, Northwestern University; Juanita Limas, University of North Carolina; Sarah Lipson, Boston University; Olivia Lubarsky, John W. Brick Foundation; and Michelle Riba, University of Michigan.

Although the reviewers listed above provided many constructive comments and suggestions, they were not asked to endorse the conclusions or recommendations of this report, nor did they see the final draft before its release. The review of this report was overseen by Antonia Villarruel, University of Pennsylvania, and Paul Gray, University of California, Berkeley. They were responsible for making certain that an independent examination of the report was carried out in accordance with the standards of the National Academies and that all review comments were carefully considered. Responsibility for the final content rests entirely with the authoring committee and the National Academies.

Contents

Summary

The United States has been struck simultaneously by three historic events: the SARS-CoV-2/COVID-19 pandemic, the associated precipitous rise in unemployment and cratering of the U.S. economy, and the killing of George Floyd, Breonna Taylor, and Ahmaud Arbery and the resulting national reckoning of the legacy of slavery, racism, and the increased awareness that people of color have different lived experiences and much more difficult lives than white people. One consequence of these three simultaneous events is an increase in anxiety and depression across the U.S. population, one that appears to be spreading and accelerating, according to a May 2020 survey conducted by Mental Health America. The rise in mental health, emotional, and behavioral issues is reflected in a marked increase in psychological distress being reported by the students at our nation's colleges and universities.[1] This is particularly true in light of the social isolation many students have experienced over the past several months, the uncertainty of how and when campuses will reopen, and existential concerns about their futures given the extreme harm the U.S. economy has suffered.

This more recent rise in student distress resulting from these three converging phenomena highlights what has long been an increasing trend in student mental health and substance use problems reported by many institutions of higher education. Data from the 2018-2019 Healthy Minds Study of more than 300,000 students at some 300 colleges and universities (Eisenberg et al., 2019), conducted before the COVID pandemic, identified the pervasiveness of this problem across

---

[1] For the purposes of this report, the term mental health will be used to refer to mental health, emotional issues, and behavioral issues. The term mental illness will be used specifically in reference to diagnosed serious mental health disorders, including depression, schizophrenia, bipolar disorder, or anxiety disorder.

the nation; almost 40 percent of students—or some 8 million postsecondary students nationwide—reported experiencing a significant mental health problem. That same survey found that 60 percent of college undergraduates have been having an increasingly difficult time accessing mental health care even before most campuses closed and instruction moved online. These increases are severely limiting the ability of the nation's colleges and universities to provide the kind of atmosphere and services needed to ensure that all students succeed and achieve their full potential. This situation also has broader implications for completion and career success of postsecondary students necessary to build and diversify the nation's workforce.

At the same time, the U.S. higher education enterprise is under tremendous financial distress, also triggered by the pandemic and resulting harm to the U.S. economy, so that finding new funds to provide additional resources for students experiencing mental health problems is proving to be problematic. Nonetheless, a December 2020 survey by the American Council on Education found that 68 percent of university presidents ranked student mental health concerns as among their most pressing issues. In fact, the top two most pressing issues for presidents across all sectors were "mental health of students" and "mental health of faculty and staff" (Turk et al., 2020). However, this understanding of the need does not always result in making student mental health concerns a priority.

While the short- and long-term outcomes of the current situation remain unknown and difficult to predict, the long-term consequences for the mental health of students in higher education are likely to be significant given the already increasing level of distress that postsecondary students were experiencing in general prior to the current challenges. Colleges and universities of all types and sizes will have to deal with this likelihood, if not for the benefit of their students and the nation that needs their graduates, then certainly for the sake of their financial situation—every student that drops out of school because of a mental health issue is a student who is not paying tuition.

In June 2019, the Substance Abuse and Mental Health Services Administration, along with the National Institute of Mental Health, National Institute on Alcohol Abuse and Alcoholism, and National Institute on Drug Abuse requested that the National Academies of Sciences, Engineering, and Medicine launch an 18-month consensus study to examine the degree to which the support systems on campuses provide services, programming, and other resources to students and the faculty, staff, and health systems with whom students interact. Under the auspices of the Board on Higher Education and Workforce, and in collaboration with the Health and Medicine Division, the National Academies appointed a committee of experts to examine the most current research and consider the ways that institutions of higher education, including community colleges, provide treatment and support for the mental health and wellbeing of undergraduate and graduate students in all fields of study. For the purposes of this report, the term mental health will be used to refer to mental health and emotional and behavioral issues. The term mental illness will be used specifically in reference to diagnosed serious mental disorders, including depression, schizophrenia, bipolar disorder, or anxiety disorder.

By contrast, wellbeing is a holistic concept referring to both physical and mental health. It includes a sense of personal safety and security, emotional support and connection, mechanisms to cope with stressors, and access to services when appropriate for short- and long-term care. The committee believes that institutions have a responsibility both to enhance the wellbeing of all students and to provide additional support to a subset of students with more severe emotional distress and mental illness. Over the course of the study, the committee:

- Identified and reviewed programs, practices, resources, and policies that institutions of higher education have developed to treat mental health issues and to support wellbeing on campuses;
- Analyzed the challenges institutions face—including financial, cultural, and human resource obstacles and methods to address these challenges;
- Investigated factors related to the funding of and access to mental health services and support for student wellbeing, such as student academic performance and campus climate;
- Examined, to the extent possible, the relationship between student mental health, wellbeing, and rates of alcohol and drug use, and recommend ways in which institutions can address substance use and its effects on campus climate; and
- Produced a consensus report with recommendations that will be broadly distributed on campuses, at professional society meetings, and in other venues.

This report presents the findings of the Committee on Supporting the Whole Student: Mental Health, Substance Abuse, and Wellbeing in Higher Education and the recommendations it developed that, if followed, would improve the delivery of mental health, wellness, and substance use services by the nation's institutions of higher education. This report also contains the committee's suggestions for further research on student wellbeing and mental health and on the delivery of such services to benefit all students. While the committee acknowledges throughout the report the potential for the COVID-19 pandemic to exacerbate mental health issues for this population, this was not the focus of the report.

The report contains some information on graduate students and medical students, but focuses primarily on undergraduate students. Even though the committee was asked to investigate mental health issues among science, technology, engineering, mathematics, and medical (STEMM) students where feasible, most of the data relevant to this study are not disaggregated by field. In addition, the issues of mental health, substance use, and wellbeing affect all students in all disciplines, as do the campus services provided to deal with them.

Similarly, although mental health issues affect students in all professional fields of study, the committee was explicitly asked by the study sponsors to focus on medical students. It has provided some information on medical students, although, given the broad scope of the study, that information is necessarily brief. In its focus on medical students, the committee acknowledges that the mental health issues facing this population frequently also apply to other health professionals, including students pursuing degrees in other health-related fields. These mental health issues have likely been exacerbated by the COVID-19 crisis, where all health professionals are facing front line stresses related to the diagnosis, treatment, and care of patients, and have been found to be at higher risk of developing psychological distress and other mental health symptoms.

WHY DOES STUDENT WELLBEING MATTER TO HIGHER EDUCATION?

Student wellbeing is foundational to academic success. One recent survey of postsecondary educators found that nearly 80 percent believed emotional wellbeing is a "very" or "extremely" important factor in student success. Studies have found that the dropout rates for students with a diagnosed mental health problem range from 43 percent to as high as 86 percent. While dealing with stress is a normal part of life, for some students, stress can adversely affect their physical, emotional, and psychological health, particularly given that adolescence and early adulthood are when most mental illnesses are first manifested. In addition to students who may develop mental health challenges during their time in postsecondary education, many students arrive on campus with a mental health problem or having experienced significant trauma in their lives, which can also negatively affect physical, emotional, and psychological wellbeing.

Although it is a time of emotional and intellectual growth, pursuing a postsecondary education at any level can be a stressful and challenging experience for many students. A variety of factors affect students' stress, including rising tuition and student debt. While these financial stressors affect many undergraduates, graduate students and medical students often face the increased burden of additional student debt after completing their undergraduate education.

First-generation students, students who graduate from underresourced high schools, non-native English speakers, and students from underrepresented groups such as students of color and sexual and gender minorities face additional challenges and stress. Moreover, the stigma of mental illness is particularly powerful for many young people in these groups, thus exacerbating the problems.

While student wellbeing is foundational to their success in postsecondary education, research shows that far too many students at all levels of their education and in all fields of study are not achieving a level of wellbeing that will enable them to thrive in an academic setting and reach their full potential.

For some students who do graduate, mental health problems are associated with breaks in their education, longer times to graduation, and lower grade-point averages. A report from the American Council on Education emphasizes the point, saying that, "the connection between mental health issues and student retention, particularly for students from historically marginalized groups, has implications for the economic wellbeing of students and institutions alike. Specifically, the negative effects of behavioral health problems on student retention suggest that institutional investments in student mental health are likely to generate both increased tuition revenues for institutions and higher earnings for students who attain a college degree" (Bruce-Sanford and Soares, 2019).

INSTITUTIONAL RESPONSIBILITY

Nearly every institution of higher education provides some version of mental health and substance use counseling and treatment services, often through a counseling and psychological services center. This institutionalized function can lead college and university leaders to assume that simply bolstering their counseling centers would be a sufficient solution to the mental health and wellbeing problems that today's students face. It is the committee's judgment, however, that counseling centers cannot and should not be expected to solve these problems alone given that the factors and forces affecting student wellbeing go well beyond the purview and resources that counseling centers can bring to bear. Rather, the committee believes institutions of higher education need to tackle two significant challenges. First, institutions must address the challenges arising from the increasing incidence of mental health problems among students in postsecondary education. Doing so will involve dedicating more resources to increase capacity for promoting wellbeing and serving those students who need help for a mental health concern or substance use. A multi-pronged approach is needed to address these challenges—including a focus on prevention, identification of high-risk students in a thoughtful way, effective community-based approaches, treatment services for identified cases, and relapse prevention and post-treatment support.

In addition, both the institutions and their faculty and staff need to address the issues within higher education institutions themselves, for example, institutional culture, that contribute to this increasing incidence of mental health and wellbeing concerns. An "all-hands" approach, one that emphasizes shared responsibility and a holistic understanding of what it means in practice to support students, is needed if institutions of higher education are to intervene from anything more than a reactive standpoint. Creating this systemic change requires that institutions examine their entire culture and environment and accept more responsibility for forming learning environments where a changing student population can thrive. Specifically, institutions of higher education need to create conditions that support mental health and help students deal with such issues when they arise. At a minimum, this requires developing a culture of support throughout the institution. The committee strongly believes that only through such a multi-pronged strategy can our nation's institutions of higher education create a supportive environment that will benefit everyone, including faculty and staff who must be active participants in this effort.

In addition to being aware of the ways in which faculty and staff might exacerbate conditions that undermine student health, these people have an underacknowledged role in promoting student wellbeing. To be successful, though, they need basic training in identifying and speaking with students who may benefit from a mental health referral. In addition, faculty need opportunities to develop skills and norms that improve their work in these areas. Faculty and staff should not be expected to act in the place of licensed counselors, but they do need to recognize issues and warning signs, empathize with students, and refer them to professionals who can help. There also is a role for undergraduate student peers and graduate teaching and research assistants in laboratories and classrooms who may be the people to whom students in crisis turn for help. The burden lies with the entire campus. Institutions should improve their infrastructure to respond to needs that arise, and their efforts must include building an institution-wide culture that values and supports student wellbeing.

MOVING FORWARD

There are no one-size-fits-all solutions to the challenges institutions of higher education are facing to meet student demand for mental health, substance use, and wellness services. A community college with an exclusively commuter student body, for example, is likely to encounter a different constellation of issues and have different resources available to deal with them when compared with a large public land-grant institution, a small private liberal arts college, or a university with a largely residential student body. The issues faced by undergraduates and graduate or professional school students can be quite different and must be recognized as such. Moreover, research has documented differences in the prevalence of symptoms and use of services across race and ethnicity, socioeconomic backgrounds, gender identities, and academic fields.

When appropriate, the committee mentions interventions designed for specific types of institutions or student populations. However, it is the committee's judgment that there are multiple proven approaches for addressing mental health and substance use issues and promoting student wellbeing and that individual institutions can best determine the approaches most appropriate to their local conditions. For that reason, the committee is not advocating for a single "ideal" that all institutions of higher education should adopt or strive toward. Instead, the committee examines five major issues confronting institutions of higher education as they work to better meet students' needs, provides examples of promising practices that have been effective at other institutions, identifies ways institutions might address barriers to progress, and points out gaps in our knowledge that future research should address. These include the following:

- Addressing institutional culture and policies
- Prioritizing mental health amid financial constraints
- Understanding the state of student mental health and wellbeing on each campus
- Assessing institutional capacity to provide needed services
- Developing faculty, staff, and student capability to support emotional wellbeing and mental health

INSTITUTIONAL CULTURE AND POLICIES

Institutions of higher education must ensure that their culture is one of acceptance of and support for those students experiencing problems with mental health and substance use. Moreover, the committee believes that ensuring this culture must start with the institution's leadership, the president and board of trustees/regents. Without institutional support and leadership, progress will be spotty, and too many students with problems will fall through the cracks. The Okanagan Charter[2] is a useful guide that can help colleges and universities embed health into all aspects of campus culture and promote collaborative action to create a health-promoting culture.

The committee acknowledges how difficult it is to change the culture of institutions of higher education, which tend to value the status quo and tradition. Nonetheless, the committee recognizes that accomplishing difficult tasks is a hallmark of the U.S. higher education enterprise. The committee believes as well that the COVID-19 pandemic and the George Floyd killing in Minneapolis have catalyzed a social movement around the disparities and racism that people of color and of low socioeconomic status experience daily in the United States. It is in the spirit of this moment that the committee believes our institutions of higher education have a special opportunity to bring together the different communities on campus to address those aspects of institutional culture that do not support, or in some instances even harm, mental health and wellbeing of all students, particularly for students from groups that have historically been excluded. At the same time, this kind of culture change, even with the highest levels of support, cannot be implemented solely by administrators, counseling center staff, and an institution's student affairs office. Rather, it requires the entire faculty, staff, and student body working together to establish a culture that recognizes the importance of attending to the demand for services that now exists, proactively addresses student mental health and substance use, supports those students who have issues, and creates an environment that supports the wellbeing of everyone

---

[2] See: https://wellbeing.ubc.ca/okanagan-charter.

on campus. Importantly, this culture change should also consider how best to engage part-time, adjunct faculty who may have significant student interaction and can support this broader culture change. Establishing a campus-wide action commission with representatives from faculty, students, staff, and administrative units, with a clear and effective leader, dedicated resources, and a clear charge to build a culture that supports student wellbeing, would be a strong first step toward promoting culture change and creating such an environment.

Aside from campus culture, institutional medical leave and re-enrollment policies can serve as barriers for students whose mental health or substance use problems are severe enough that they lead the student to withdraw from school at least temporarily. Many institutions have a limit to how long a student's leave of absence can last before having to reapply for readmission, and withdrawal from school can affect students' financial aid. However, students with disabilities, including those related to mental health (the most common type) and substance use, have the right to reasonable accommodations for their disability according to the Americans with Disabilities Act. Such accommodations include extra time on exams or assignments, the ability to withdraw from specific classes, and leaves of absence that allow for re-enrollment.

An important step toward creating an integrated approach to supporting students would be to establish a closer collaboration between academic affairs and student affairs. This step has been shown to help increase the chances for students with mental health or substance use issues to access services and succeed in school.

Considering Student Voices and Perspectives

Colleges and universities need to listen carefully to the voices and perspectives of the students themselves, both to understand how the institutions contribute to student stress as well as to understand how to change the campus culture and environment in order to minimize that stress and promote emotional wellness on campus. Students are often keenly aware of what needs to change in their environment and what is needed to support their own and others' mental health. In addition, they are often the first to witness unusual or troubling behavior in their peers and are often the first line of support. A concerted effort on the part of administrative leadership, faculty, and staff is needed to create both formal and informal ways to include students in actions to change the culture on campus, revise policies that contribute to emotional and financial distress or threaten physical safety, combat systemic racism, publicize widely the availability of mental health resources, develop training to faculty and staff, and offer multiple ways for individual students to seek help. Most of these efforts will benefit the entire community.

PRIORITIZING MENTAL HEALTH AMID
FINANCIAL CONSTRAINTS

Economic pressures, including increased operating costs, and greater market competition, have been on the rise for U.S. institutions of higher education for well over a decade. A 2014 survey of college and university board chairs and presidents, for example, found that 77 percent believe the financial stability of higher education is moving in the wrong direction (Selingo, 2015). This situation has been made worse by the COVID-19 pandemic that forced colleges and universities to effectively close their campuses for educational purposes and move to online instruction. The report notes, too, that the cost of student services and student facilities, such as campus counseling centers, represent a major concern to university presidents.

All of this is to say that academic budgets at all types of institutions are already constrained, a situation that makes creating new programs or embarking on new initiatives challenging for academic leaders. However, the assumption that bolstering the capabilities of the counseling and psychological services centers and creating other programs aimed at improving student wellbeing will simply create another major financial burden for colleges and universities with no tangible benefits is not necessarily true. Colleges and universities lose revenues when students drop out because of mental health or substance use problems. In fact, the Healthy Minds Network, which has developed a return on investment tool, has calculated that a counseling center treating 500 students a year will help an average of 30 students remain enrolled in college and increase tuition revenues by $1.2 million. In addition, those 30 students' lifetime earnings would increase by an estimated $3 million (Lipson and Roy, 2015). Other research has shown that counseling services have a positive impact on retention.

Another approach colleges and universities can take is to start or expand billing of insurance companies for services rendered, something that less than 5 percent of institutions currently do, in part because the time, expense, and human resources needed to create the infrastructure to bill insurance companies may be beyond the capabilities of smaller institutions and community colleges. Colleges and universities that do bill insurance have not completely solved the demand/supply concern, highlighting that this problem is a broader institutional priority question. In addition, for colleges and universities that do not mandate that students have insurance coverage, there will be uninsured students who would not be able to afford services that require payment. The insurance reimbursement issue is further complicated by state insurance regulations that need to be changed.

UNDERSTANDING THE STATE OF STUDENT MENTAL
HEALTH AND WELLBEING ON EACH CAMPUS

Data on mental health and substance use in students can be challenging to interpret for a number of reasons. These data are drawn from different groups of students, including those seeking mental health services in counseling centers, subjects of targeted surveys on specific problems, higher education students in general, and broader segments of an age-equivalent population in and outside academia. Also, multiple methods are used in data collection, with varying strengths and limitations.

Much of the information on the incidence of mental health and substance use problems among students is based on self-reports from general population surveys, not actual clinical evaluations. This approach provides an economical way to collect data from entire student populations, but it typically relies on brief screens that are correlated with but not equivalent to clinical evaluations.

Data from clinical settings are drawn from students who use mental health services from a counseling center in order to be evaluated or receive treatment. These data have the potential to characterize the full sub-population, and they include assessments by clinicians instead of or in addition to self-reported symptoms. They are, however, limited to those who use clinical services and therefore do not represent students who are not accessing those services.

No single data point or source of data is capable of conveying the complexity of mental health and substance use problems among students. Multiple approaches and methodologies contribute to a richer understanding of the issues, but the strengths and limitations of each approach need to be taken into account in forming conclusions about the prevalence of mental health and substance use issues in higher education.

INSTITUTIONAL CAPACITY TO PROVIDE NEEDED SERVICES

Once an institution has determined the extent of mental health and substance use issues among its students, it needs to determine whether it has the resources available—either on campus or in the local community—to support student mental health and to provide adequate care for those students suffering from those conditions. The great majority of university presidents surveyed indicated that they provide mental health services for their students, and another 12 percent are considering different options to address student mental health and substance use in light of COVID-19. However, there is not enough capacity in terms of mental health and substance use professionals for the general population, let alone to help every student who needs help, whether in a campus setting or via a community resource. According to the Health Resources and Services Administration, this situation is projected to get worse, not better, in the years ahead.

Possible partial solutions include increasing the use of teletherapy, enabling peer-to-peer support initiatives, and turning to the community, including university and local health services, to increase capacity, particularly for students with more serious mental health issues. In addition, institutions of higher education should initiate campus-wide efforts to raise mental health awareness and to prevent suicide, which they can do through mandatory orientations for new faculty, staff, and students. Some institutions of higher education have established mental health teams. The Jed Foundation highlights Campus Behavioral Intervention Teams (BIT) that "promote student, faculty and staff success and campus safety by facilitating the identification and support of individuals who demonstrate behaviors that may be early warning signs of possible troubled, disruptive or violent behavior" (Jed Foundation, 2016).

In whatever way an institution decides to increase its capacity to address student mental health and substance use problems, it should ensure that available resources can support diverse student populations. The Equity in Mental Health Framework, for example, is an accessible resource for schools seeking to promote mental health and wellbeing among Black, Indigenous, and people of color, as well as students with other identities, including sexual and gender minorities.

DEVELOPING FACULTY, STAFF, AND STUDENT CAPABILITY TO SUPPORT EMOTIONAL WELLBEING AND MENTAL HEALTH

It takes everyone on campus to contribute to an environment that fosters student wellbeing, protects students from developing mental health and substance use issues, and helps facilitate access to services that would benefit them. Faculty and staff, including graduate student teaching assistants and residence hall assistants, have an important role to play in this effort given that they are in regular contact with students. At some institutions, particularly community colleges, faculty are likely to be the only members with whom students interact on a regular basis. The culture of many institutions of higher education and their incentive structures—at both the disciplinary levels and within the specific workplaces where research is carried out—have been poorly aligned with creating inclusive environments, and faculty have not been held accountable nor rewarded for creating an environment that supports wellbeing among students, whether in the classroom or the laboratory.

Faculty members can, however, play a significant role if appropriately trained. Periodic training on mental health issues as well as ways to help reduce stress and promote wellbeing in classrooms is needed for faculty and staff, particularly for those who directly support students, including graduate teaching and research assistants and postdoctoral researchers. Training related to mental health should include understanding of racial/ethnic, class, and other disparities in experiences of and attitudes toward mental health treatment. Most importantly, faculty should be taught how to identify and respond to students in distress and feel confident to help them access services. What the committee envisions is an approach that would provide faculty with basic training in four areas:

- how to identify, initiate conversations with, and refer students who may be having problems with mental health or substance use;

- how to make learning environments inclusive and supportive of student wellbeing;
- how to model preventive strategies and coping skills in class; and
- how to improve mentorship skills and pedagogical skills so that relationships and instruction support wellbeing.

RECOMMENDATIONS

The committee presents 10 sets of recommendations, all in Chapter 5, to improve the ability to provide wellbeing, mental health and substance use services for students that meet the increasing demands for such services. The recommendations are as follows:

RECOMMENDATION 5-1
Institutional leaders, starting with the president and board of trustees or regents, should articulate the importance of creating a culture of wellbeing on their campus, one that recognizes the range of individual behaviors and community norms that affect wellbeing, acknowledges the magnitude of mental health and substance use issues on campus, addresses the stigma associated with mental illness and substance use disorders, and provides a range of resources to support students with different levels of need.

RECOMMENDATION 5-2
Leadership from all segments of the campus community is needed to promote a culture of wellbeing.
- Institutions of higher education should establish and/or maintain a team or teams that involves all sectors of the institution's community that coordinates, reviews, and addresses mental health, substance use, and wellbeing concerns.
- Any approach should have shared responsibility for addressing issues that negatively affect student wellbeing, a clear leadership structure and mandate, appropriate access to financial resources, and a charge to develop and implement an action plan to promote and support student wellbeing.

RECOMMENDATION 5-3
Institutions should ensure their leave of absence and reenrollment policies and practices will accommodate the needs of students experiencing mental health and substance use problems and the time needed for effective treatment and recovery.
- Institutions should implement methods to reduce and/or alleviate financial burden on students related to medical leave and other issues related to course completion.

- Academic affairs and student affairs units should develop collaborations to share information appropriately, while also respecting a student's right to private/confidential treatment, in order to support students at the intersection of mental health and academic concerns.

RECOMMENDATION 5-4
Institutions of higher education and the government agencies that support them should increase the priority given to funding for campus and community mental health and substance use services.

- National, state, and local funders of higher education should incentivize colleges and universities to effectively provide support for students' mental health and substance use problems.
- In their budgets, hiring, programming, expectations for serving students, and assessment/evaluation activities, institutions should make mental health a higher priority on campus. They should also work more directly with state and local governments, where relevant, to help bring this about.
- To ensure that mental health and emotional wellness services are prioritized, institutions should consider reallocating existing institutional funds to support counseling centers, support the increased use of online mental health services (when appropriate), and support data collection on the need for and use of mental health services by students.
- Institutions should actively collaborate with local health care services and facilities and community providers, for example, by considering hiring staff to help students navigate and manage off-campus services.
- States should modify insurance laws or regulations, or provide administrative guidance, to enable institutions to use general funds and/or designated health fees for expenses that are not covered by students' personal insurance.

RECOMMENDATION 5-5
Institutions of higher education should work with insurance companies and health plans and federal, state and local regulators to remove barriers to seeking reimbursement for student mental health and substance use costs for covered students.

- Insurance companies should keep up with market rates for reimbursement to incentivize more providers to accept insurance carried by students, support providers from institutions of higher education in becoming paneled quickly, and communicate and improve the confidentiality measures in place to dependent subscribers between the ages of 18-26 to ensure that they can seek services using their parents' insurance and be afforded the confidentiality they are entitled to receive.
- States should modify insurance laws or regulations, or provide administrative guidance, to enable institutions to use general funds and/or designated

health fees for expenses that are not covered by students' personal insurance for charges incurred at student health and counseling services. This is commonly referred to as a secondary payor provision in coordination of benefits.

RECOMMENDATION 5-6
Institutions of higher education should conduct a regular (preferably at least every 2 years) assessment that addresses student mental health, substance use, wellbeing, and campus climate. The data generated from these assessments should be compared to peer institution data (as available for disaggregation). Analysts should create a data collection system that allows for disaggregation by unit, program level, and student identities. This assessment should include the extent that students are aware of and know how to access available resources, both on campus and in the local community, to address students' mental health and substance use problems.
- At the end of the academic year, institutions should review the many data points collected about their clinical trends and utilization as a way to understand how resources on campus can be used most effectively. These data would include the percentage of students who received treatment at the institution, the percentage that went outside of the institution for treatment, and the percentage of students that report needing help but did not seek or receive it, and should be further analyzed across demographic and identity groups.
- Funding agencies and private organizations should provide grants to under-resourced institutions, notably community colleges, historically Black colleges and universities, and tribal colleges and universities, to collect, analyze, and share data with the goal of implementing findings.

RECOMMENDATION 5-7
Institutions of higher education should work to ensure students have access to high-quality mental health and substance use treatment services. These services can be provided either on campus or in the local community. In order to ensure students have this access:
- After conducting a needs assessment and reviewing available mental health resources on and off campus, institutional leadership should attempt to measure and define the "gap" between need for mental health care and capacity for care. That gap should then be examined for solutions from multiple angles but especially long-term funding strategies and/or community partnerships.
- Institutions of higher education should design and implement culturally responsive services and programs to serve the needs and identities of all students.

- Colleges and universities should make behaviorally focused mental health services more readily available in primary care settings to facilitate students' access to care and improve coordination between mental health and primary care providers, both on campus and in telehealth services.
- Institutions of higher education should create collaborative relationships in the community that will increase clinician diversity to better serve diverse student populations.
- If counseling centers rely on community-based resources to meet the mental health needs of their students, they should consider investing in case managers/resource navigators to help students connect with these community-based resources.
- Institutions can make wide use of telehealth options for those populations and situations for which it is appropriate.

RECOMMENDATION 5-8
Provide and require faculty training on how to create an inclusive and healthy learning environment.
- Provide and require faculty training about how to recognize students in distress and appropriately refer them to appropriate care.
- Provide mentor training, starting in graduate school, for all faculty, recognizing that good mentorship practices serve as a protective factor for student mental health.

RECOMMENDATION 5-9
As a part of formal orientation to college life, all students should participate in structured opportunities to learn about individual wellbeing and the cultivation of a healthy, respectful campus climate. This orientation should also include material on how to develop resilience in the face of inevitable challenges they will experience both in college and in life.
- To enable students' self-awareness and resilience, training should acknowledge how behaviors such as sleep, nutrition, exercise, social media, and work can be both levers for wellbeing as well as affected by wellbeing.
- Training should also include information on how to recognize and address implicit bias, and about the essential role students themselves play in creating a community that supports each other's wellbeing.
- The institution should also periodically offer refresher or "booster" training on these issues.
- Institutions should regularly and widely provide guidance to students and faculty on mental health resources available on campus and in the community.

RECOMMENDATION 5-10
Institutions of higher education should recognize that there is no single approach to promoting wellbeing and dealing with mental health and substance use problems that will be appropriate for all student populations.

- Support services should be tailored to the unique histories, circumstances, and needs of individual student populations.
- Support services should recognize and respond to the fact that many students from diverse populations will have experienced interpersonal racism, systemic racism, and implicit bias both before and during their time in higher education.

1

Introduction

Postsecondary students, from those attending community colleges to professional and graduate students, are reporting rising rates of anxiety, depression, suicidal thoughts, trauma, and substance use (see Box 1-1) (Xiao et al., 2017).[1] Many undergraduate students experience the onset of mental health and substance use problems or an exacerbation of their symptoms during this critical developmental stage (Pedrelli et al., 2015). These increases call for substantial improvements in how the nation's institutions of higher education engage with students, and for institutions to recognize how their policies, practices, and cultures can affect and support student mental health[2] and wellbeing more broadly (Posselt, 2018b). Treating mental illness at this stage in an individual's development is key to lessening the potential for chronic mental conditions. More purposeful engagement by postsecondary institutions can help ameliorate some of the stresses unique to higher education that go beyond, for example, just being a young adult, veteran, or working adult returning to campus.

While mental health and substance use problems have increased significantly over the past decades, there is now heightened awareness about how the crises currently disrupting American life are exacerbating these problems. The COVID-19

---

[1] Much of the information on the incidence of mental health and substance use problems among students comes from self-reports and not actual diagnoses. Self-report data can be inaccurate and may not in fact reflect well the true incidence of those issues among students in higher education (Dang et al., 2020). Chapter 6 discusses research needed to address this limitation.

[2] The committee has chosen to use the term "mental health" to refer collectively to mental health, the absence of or, at least, low levels of substance use, and wellbeing, and the term "mental illness" to refer to diagnosed, serious mental health problems such as depression, bipolar disorder, and anxiety disorder.

BOX 1-1
Indicators of Mental Health Issues in Postsecondary Education

Data from the 2018-2019 Healthy Minds Study[a] of more than 300,000 students at some 300 colleges and universities (Eisenberg et al., 2019), conducted before the COVID pandemic, illustrate the challenges that postsecondary students report experiencing prior to the pandemic:

- Almost 40 percent of students—or some 8 million postsecondary students nationwide—reported experiencing a significant mental health problem.
- Major depression[b] affected 18 percent of the students surveyed, while another 18 percent were found to have moderate depression, up from 8 percent with major depression and 14 percent with moderate depression in 2007.
- Severe anxiety affected 14 percent of the students surveyed compared to 6 percent in 2017. Another 17 percent of students reported symptoms of moderate anxiety.
- Eating disorders affected 10 percent of the students surveyed, a near doubling since 2013, and 34 percent expressed an elevated level of eating concerns.
- Suicidal ideation during the past year was reported by 14 percent of the students surveyed, with 6 percent planning suicide at some point, 2 percent making a suicide attempt, and 24 percent inflicting non-suicidal self-injury. In 2007, those figures were 6 percent, 1.5 percent, 0.6 percent, and 14 percent, respectively.
- One in 10 students indicated that they had experienced sexual assault in the past year, with 72 percent of these students screening positive for one or more significant mental health problem, compared to 47 percent of students without a history of sexual assault.
- Some 20 percent of students felt that emotional or mental difficulties had hurt their academic performance for six days or more over the previous four weeks.
- Based on students' self-perceived successes in areas such as relationships, self-esteem, purpose, and optimism, only 40 percent of students were judged to have positive mental health or be flourishing, compared to 57 percent in 2012.
- Marijuana use among postsecondary students increased between 2007 and 2019, rising from 14 percent of students reporting the use of marijuana over the previous 30 days to 24 percent.
- Binge drinking decreased between 2007 and 2019, falling from 43 percent of students who reported binge drinking more than one time during the year to 37 percent, although the volume of drinking increased (HMN, 2020).

---

[a] The Healthy Minds Network has administered an annual web-based survey of undergraduate and graduate student mental health–related issues since 2007. More information about the network and the annual survey are available at https://healthymindsnetwork.org/data/ (accessed March 24, 2020).

[b] The National Institute of Mental Health defines major depression, also called clinical depression, as a mental health disorder characterized by persistently depressed mood or loss of interest in activities, causing significant impairment in daily life.

pandemic is one. Institutions of higher education have closed campuses, moved instruction online, and mandated physical distancing. This, in turn, has caused substantial disruptions in the lives of the nation's college students, including loss of income, anxieties about their future educational and job prospects, and disconnection from the social interactions that are a normal part of college and young adult life. Indeed, a Kaiser Family Foundation survey conducted during the spring 2020 outbreak found that 45 percent of adults believed the pandemic affected their mental health, and 19 percent reported that the pandemic had a major effect on it (Kirzinger et al., 2020; Panchal et al., 2020). A weekly survey conducted by Mental Health America found a 19 percent increase in screening for clinical anxiety was already occurring during the first weeks of February and a further 12 percent increase was seen in the first two weeks of March (MHA, 2020a). The National Institute on Drug Abuse has issued an alert that the pandemic could hit some populations with substance use disorders particularly hard (NIDA, 2020d). According to Kaiser Family Foundation researchers, "the pandemic is likely to have both long- and short-term implications for mental health and substance use. Those with mental illness and substance use disorders pre-pandemic, and those newly affected, will likely require mental health and substance use services" (Panchal et al., 2020).

Surveys administered later in the pandemic have suggested these same trends are present at the same or even higher levels in college students (see Box 1-2) (HMN and ACHA, 2020). An April 2020 survey by the American Council of Education found that 41 percent of university presidents ranked student mental health concerns as one of the five most pressing issues facing their institutions (Turk et al., 2020a). In addition, roughly 1,700 respondents to another survey by Active Minds said the pandemic negatively affected their mental health and 20 percent said their mental health had significantly worsened during the pandemic (Active Minds, 2020). More than half of the students surveyed said they would not know where to go if they or someone they knew needed professional mental health services immediately. The rise in the prevalence of mental health problems is not unique to college student populations; the prevalence is rising in adolescent and young adult populations overall.

The second major crisis currently afflicting American life is the economic turmoil that has accompanied the COVID-19 outbreak. Colleges and universities are facing unprecedented financial challenges resulting from the loss of tuition revenues, uncertainty about future enrollment, and the costs of preparing their campuses to allow students, faculty, and staff to return safely, or absent that, preparing to deliver coursework online (Startz, 2020). Faculty, staff, and students alike are experiencing loss of work and wages, which also increase the risks of experiencing mental health and substance use problems. This may be particularly true for students coming from communities of color or lower socioeconomic backgrounds, whom the pandemic has affected disproportionately.

BOX 1-2
The COVID-19 Pandemic, Mental Health, and Higher Education

While the long-lasting impact of COVID-19 on higher education will continue to interest researchers in the coming years, many colleges and universities are seeking ways to understand the immediate impact and ways to mitigate the negative stress on students. The end of the 2019-2020 academic year was met with early closures of campuses, a transition to virtual classrooms, and the loss of graduations and other landmark events. As leadership, faculty and staff, students and families, and the surrounding communities looked to the start of the 2020-2021 academic year, a new set of questions emerged: Will students be allowed back on campus and when will a final determination be made? What are the safety and risk factors? What happens if the situation gets worse?

Although there is some disagreement about the magnitude of the problem, there is agreement that the pandemic has exacerbated an already large problem. For example, the Healthy Minds Study and the American College Health Association's report *The Impact of COVID-19 on College Student Wellbeing* provided data from 14 campuses.[a]

Main findings include:
- 23.3 percent of students reported that it was "much more difficult" and 36.8 reported that it was "somewhat more difficult" to access mental health care.
- 26.4 percent reported their financial situation to be "a lot more stressful" and 39.6 percent reported it to be "somewhat more stressful."
- Compared to fall 2019, self-reported rates of depression increased, substance use decreased, and more students reported that mental health negatively impacted their academic performance. Overall, students reported lower levels of psychological wellbeing in March–May 2020 in comparison to fall 2019, however, they also indicated higher levels of resiliency. The survey also indicates concerns about the future, from how long will the pandemic last (64.8 percent very or extremely concerned) and people they care about contracting COVID-19 (64.4 percent were very or extremely concerned). As the economic environment, labor market, and social unrest continue to affect all individuals living in the United States, additional data gathering and research on the impact of students will help colleges and universities understand the ways to provide support and address mental health for those enrolled. See Chapter 6 for additional detail on the research agenda.

_____

[a] A total of 14 colleges and universities participated in the two studies between March and May 2020: seven for Healthy Minds Study (HMS) and seven for American College Health Association National College Health Assessment (ACHA-NCHA). They included one two-year college. Thirteen of the campuses have 10,000 or more students, and one has less than 2,500 students.

Finally, the nation is facing a third crisis with significant effects on the physical and mental health of students of color and other historically underrepresented groups highlighted by the mass demonstrations and calls for racial justice following the murders of George Floyd, Breonna Taylor, and Ahmaud Arbery. In response to these murders, institutions of higher education, along with many other institutions and structures in our nation, have a growing recognition of the work that must be done to address systemic racism and dismantle inequities. The national energy to address racism and racial disparities raises the imperative to address issues that disproportionately affect students of color and those from other underserved populations so that all students can thrive during and after their years in higher education.

STUDENT WELLBEING IS FOUNDATIONAL FOR SUCCESS

The concept of wellbeing, according to the Centers for Disease Control and Prevention (CDC), refers to "the presence of positive emotions and moods (e.g., contentment or happiness), the absence of negative emotions (e.g., depression or anxiety), satisfaction with life, fulfillment, and positive functioning" (Andrews and Withey, 1976; CDC, 2018; Diener, 2000). Student wellbeing is foundational to academic success.

The CDC and other leading public health organizations argue that wellbeing has mental, emotional, physical, spiritual, social, financial, and other dimensions that, individually and collectively, impact a variety of outcomes of concern to colleges and universities. Student wellbeing is about more than just having happy students: a large body of research has shown that mental health challenges significantly affect academic achievement and graduation rates in postsecondary education (Mojtabai et al., 2015).

Just as wellbeing is a foundational element for students' success in day-to-day life, it is equally important for degree completion. However, judging from the figures cited in Box 1-1, far too many postsecondary students are not experiencing a level of wellbeing that will enable them to thrive in an academic setting and reach their full potential.

While dealing with stress is a normal part of life, for some students stress can adversely affect their physical, emotional, and psychological health (Hartley, 2011; Shankar and Park, 2016). Moreover, studies have found that dropout rates for students with a diagnosable mental health problem range from 43 percent (Breslau et al., 2008) to as high as 86 percent (Collins and Mowbray, 2005). This risk is particularly relevant for institutions of higher education given that adolescence and early adulthood is when most mental illnesses are first experienced (American Psychiatric Association, 2018). Mental health issues may appear in children and adolescents. A literature review of related studies found evidence of mental health problems in adolescents, with increases being more prevalent in girls than boys (Haidt and Twenge, 2019). Thus, many undergraduate and graduate students arrive on campus with an undiagnosed mental illness that becomes salient during their years as students.

Addressing the Mental Health Challenges of Students

In addition to students who may develop mental health challenges during their time in postsecondary education, growing numbers of students arrive on campus with a current mental health or substance use problem or having experienced significant trauma in their lives that intensifies the stress response. Managing that stress response can sap attentional energy—the "bandwidth" necessary for academic success—negatively affect their physical, emotional, and psychological wellbeing (Verschelden, 2017). Stress, such as the isolation students are experiencing during the COVID pandemic, can be a major factor causing relapse and should be factored into plans for dealing with substance use, particularly in the post-pandemic period of full reopening.

Although it is a time of emotional and intellectual growth, pursuing a postsecondary education, whether at a community college, baccalaureate institution, or in a graduate or professional degree program, can be a stressful and challenging experience for many students and negatively affect wellbeing (Larcombe et al., 2016; Liu et al, 2019).

This can be particularly true for students from historically excluded groups such as students who are Black, Indigenous, and people of color, first-generation students; students who graduate from under-resourced high schools, non-native English speakers; students with disabilities; and sexual and gender minorities. While education has been characterized as the great equalizer, institutions of higher education have hardly been immune from the systemic inequalities and racism that have constrained equal opportunity, adding further stressors to students' academic resilience. Awareness of how students experience stressors within educational environments is critical, whether it is in activating effects of past trauma, revealing undiagnosed mental health issues, or navigating social and institutional mechanisms of privilege and equity. In the general population, studies have indicated that, for some underrepresented minorities, mental illness can be seen as highly stigmatizing and can result in lower treatment-seeking, depending on the context (Gary, 2005; NMHA, 1998; Ward et al., 2014). However, this has not been found to be the case for college students of color. In a study examining enrollment and counseling center service utilization data at 66 universities, Hayes et al. (2011) found no difference in utilization of counseling services between ethnic minority students and European American students. In fact, the authors found that "among students of color, utilization of campus counseling services was predicted by greater psychological distress, less family support, and a history of previous psychological problems." The authors also found that the ethnic composition of the student body, as well as the ethnic composition of the counseling center staff, predicted the likelihood that students would seek counseling services. For example, the higher the percentage of African American therapists at a university counseling center, the greater the percentage of African American students who sought services. Some programs that address these issues, including the stigma of mental health for all students as well as underrepresented minority students, are described in Chapter 3.

Results from the Healthy Minds study have shown that across all types of postsecondary institutions and fields of study, students reporting mental health problems were twice as likely as other students to drop out of school before completing their degree (Eisenberg, Golberstein, and Gollust, 2009). Even for those students who do graduate, mental health problems can be associated with breaks in their education (Arria et al., 2013), longer times to graduation, and lower grade point averages. In addition, a Microsoft/Economist Intelligence Unit survey found that 79 percent of postsecondary educators believe that emotional wellbeing is a "very" or "extremely" important factor in student academic success. Seventy percent of those surveyed believed that emotional wellbeing has become more important for student success than when they started their careers (Green, 2019).

Further along in their intellectual and career development, graduate and professional students' mental health are growing concerns, too. It has been reported that the rates of mental health problems in graduate students is six times that of the general population (Evans et al., 2018). A 2014 report from the University of California, Berkeley, found that 43 to 46 percent of bioscience graduate students reported that they were depressed (Panger, Tryon, and Smith, 2014). A more recent survey of nearly 2,300 doctoral and master's degree students across all fields found that graduate students were four times more likely to suffer from depression and anxiety than a member of the general public in the same age group (Evans et al., 2018). Greater than 40 percent of graduate students surveyed had moderate to severe anxiety, and nearly 40 percent had moderate to severe depression. Similarly, a 2014 survey of medical students found that 58 percent screened positive for depression and nearly 75 percent reported a high or intermediate level of emotional exhaustion (Dyrbye et al., 2014). In other survey data from 89 institutions, there was considerable variation in the rates of depression and anxiety by field of study and social identities in the graduate and professional student population, suggesting the need for targeted attention and efforts at this level (Posselt, 2016). See Box 1-3 for key definitions related to mental health and substance use.

THE CASE FOR SHARED RESPONSIBILITY

The goal of postsecondary education is to equip students with the knowledge and degree credentials that will enable them to be productive members of society. Hence, it will undoubtedly further an institution's academic mission to increase student degree completion rates and foster a higher level of student performance and learning via a campus-wide focus on student mental health and wellbeing. One recent study found that 25 percent of students who dropped out of college

---

BOX 1-3
Select Definitions Related to Mental Illness
and Substance Use Disorders

Early intervention is defined as "diagnosing and treating a mental illness when it first develops" (NIMH, 2020g).

Any mental illness (AMI) is defined as "a mental, behavioral, or emotional disorder. AMI can vary in impact, ranging from no impairment to mild, moderate, and even severe impairment (e.g., individuals with serious mental illness as defined below)" (NIMH, 2020h).

Serious mental illness (SMI) is defined as a "mental, behavioral, or emotional disorder resulting in serious functional impairment, which substantially interferes with or limits one or more major life activities. The burden of mental illnesses is particularly concentrated among those who experience disability due to SMI" (NIMH, 2020h).

Substance use disorder (SUD) is defined as a "medical illness caused by disordered use of a substance or substances. According to the fifth edition of the *Diagnostic and Statistical Manual of Mental Disorders* (DSM-5), SUDs are characterized by clinically significant impairments in health, social function, and impaired control over substance use and are diagnosed through assessing cognitive, behavioral, and psychological symptoms. An SUD can range from mild to severe" (NIDA, 2020b).

Treatment for mental illnesses usually consists of therapy, medication, or a combination of the two. Treatment can be given in person or through a phone or computer (telehealth) (NIMH, 2020a).

Wellbeing has a variety of definitions, but for the purposes of this report, wellbeing is a holistic concept referring to both physical and mental health. Mental wellbeing includes a sense of personal safety and security, emotional support and connection, mechanisms to cope with stressors, and access to services when appropriate for short- and long-term care.

---

with a grade point average less than 3.0 screened positive for at least one mental illness. Another study showed that some 30 percent of college students suffering from depression will drop out of school (Douce and Keeling, 2014). For students from historically underserved groups who may have been underdiagnosed, there may be higher levels of undetected psychiatric problems that increase students' risk of developing mental health problems while on campus. Attending to the multifactorial dynamics in mental health and wellbeing requires paying attention to the interplay between historical factors in psychiatric diagnosis by race and ethnicity (Chen et al., 2019).

A report from the American Council on Education emphasizes the point, saying, "the connection between mental health issues and student retention, particularly for students from historically underserved groups, has implications for the economic wellbeing of students and institutions alike. Specifically, the negative effects of mental health and substance use problems on student retention suggest that institutional investments in student mental health are likely to generate both increased tuition revenues for institutions and higher earnings for students who attain a college degree" (Lipson, Lattie, and Eisenberg, 2019). As this report discusses in Chapter 5, investing resources to address student mental health issues and foster student wellbeing can have a sizable return on investment, both for the institution and society at large (Eisenberg, Golberstein, and Hunt, 2009). Additional motivations for postsecondary institutions to promote student wellbeing include transient and repeated relocation away from natural support systems, a rising awareness that higher education's own culture can compromise wellbeing, and evidence that healthier academic communities are more productive and creative.

Virtually every institution of higher education provides some sort of mental health counseling, typically through a counseling and psychological services center. This institutionalized function, though usually underfunded to provide all of the mental health needs for matriculating students, can lead college and university leaders to assume that simply bolstering their counseling centers could be an acceptable solution to mental health problems that today's students face. It is the committee's judgment, however, that counseling centers cannot and should not be expected to solve these problems alone, given that the factors and forces affecting student wellbeing go well beyond the purview and resources that counseling centers can bring to bear. Moreover, the committee believes institutions of higher education need to tackle two significant challenges. First, they must address the challenges arising from the increasing incidence of mental health and substance use issues among students in postsecondary education. In addition, both the institutions and their faculty and staff need to address the issues within higher education institutions themselves that contribute to this increasing incidence. A primary factor in dealing with these issues is the need for institutions to address the inadequate resources currently assigned in most places to counseling centers after decades of mental health interventions designed to identify and refer students to treatment.

Another driver for colleges and universities to improve the mental health and substance use services they offer is accreditation. The Department of Education delegated to accreditation organizations the responsibility to evaluate and certify that colleges and universities are providing quality education and value to the public. In fact, accreditation approval is a key factor in universities and colleges qualifying for federal funding for research and education. These accreditation organizations, such as the Higher Learning Commission, several regional accrediting bodies, and others, have recently strengthened their standards for higher education institutions to track and improve student outcomes in the areas of retention, completion rates, job placement, and graduate school placement, all outcomes that are negatively affected when student mental health issues are not addressed. For example, the new 2020 Higher Learning Commission accreditation standards state, "the institution pursues educational improvement through goals and strategies that improve retention, persistence and completion rates in its degree programs (Standard 4.C.)" and "the institution implements its plans to systematically improve its operations and student outcomes (Standard 5.C.6)."[3]

An "all hands" approach, one that emphasizes shared responsibility and a holistic understanding of what it means in practice to support students, is needed if institutions of higher education are to intervene from anything more than a reactive standpoint. Creating this systemic change requires that institutions examine the entire culture and environment of the institution and accept more responsibility for creating learning environments where a changing student population can thrive. Specifically, creating conditions that support mental health and helping students deal with mental health and substance use issues when they arise, including helping them access adequate professional help, requires mobilizing commitment and actions by the entire institution. The committee strongly believes that only through such a multi-pronged strategy (see Chapter 5) can our nation's institutions of higher education create a supportive environment that will benefit everyone, including faculty and staff who must be active participants in this effort.

In addition to being aware of the ways in which they might exacerbate conditions that undermine student health, faculty have an underacknowledged role in promoting student mental health. This is not to say that faculty should become professional counselors or therapists. They are front-line workers, however, and therefore should have basic training in identifying and speaking with students who may benefit from an intervention for a mental health concern or other stressor, such as food or housing insecurity. Faculty should know about the main offices on campus that provide students with support for basic needs and mental health, as well as those that offer wellbeing programs. Faculty also need training to understand how their own teaching, mentoring, supervision, and lab leadership affect their student's mental health, and they need opportunities to develop skills and norms that improve their work in these areas (NASEM, 2019b). Again, faculty should not act in the place of trained counselors, but they do need to promote a healthy learning environment, recognize issues, empathize with students, and refer them to professionals who can help.

It is the responsibility of the entire university community (administrators, faculty, and staff)—not solely students and those who treat them—to consider student perspectives and incorporate their suggestions to create an environment of health, safety, inclusiveness, respect, and wellbeing.

Institutional leaders should strive toward wellness of academia as a whole, rather than just focusing on students. The culture of academia can be a hostile

---

[3] The criteria for accreditation from the Higher Learning Commission can be found at https://www.hlcommission.org/Policies/revised-criteria-for-accreditation.html (accessed August 3, 2020).

environment for students and can create or exacerbate mental health issues. Institutional leadership must consider that asking students to change their own circumstances without institutional help is beyond what can be reasonably expected, particularly for students who come from historically marginalized or excluded populations.

Systemic racism in the United States has a major impact on students' sense of safety, wellbeing, and mental health, particularly but not only for students of color. Although the impact of systemic racism on student wellbeing and mental health warrants an entirely separate study, the committee emphasizes that it is critical for institutions to examine the extent to which racism affects and threatens students and all other members of the academic community. Listening to the voices of students, staff, and professors who have been the target of racism is the only way to learn how pervasive it is. As a recent report notes, "racial trauma-informed leadership prioritizes listening, demonstrates empathy towards injustices and inequalities experienced by students of color, and creates and adapts resources that respond to their mental health needs" (Steve Fund, 2020).

Institutions should look especially carefully at policies that affect the academic and social environment, including alcohol and other drug policies and policies on sexual harassment and assault, as well as those that govern student organizations such as fraternities and sororities and their off-campus venues.

In summary, to realize long-term, widescale improvements in student wellbeing, institutions should both *improve their infrastructure* to respond to needs that arise and *improve the qualities of environments* in which students already work and learn. They need to become more proactive and less reactive in ensuring a climate that promotes wellness for everyone on campus.

BACKGROUND OF THE REPORT

To understand how the culture of a given institution of higher education affects student wellbeing and can trigger student mental health problems or exacerbate existing ones, and to identify approaches that institutions can adopt to foster student wellbeing and help those students who are having difficulties, the National Academies of Sciences, Engineering, and Medicine launched an 18-month consensus study in June 2019. Under the auspices of the Board on Higher Education and Workforce, and in collaboration with the Health and Medicine Division, the National Academies appointed a committee of experts to examine the most current research and consider the ways that institutions of higher education, including community colleges, provide treatment and support for the mental health and wellbeing of undergraduate and graduate students in all fields of study. For the purposes of this report, the term mental health will be used to refer to mental health and emotional and behavioral issues. The term mental illness will be used specifically in reference to diagnosed serious mental disorders, including depression, schizophrenia, bipolar disorder, or anxiety disorder.

By contrast, wellbeing is a holistic concept referring to both physical and mental health. Mental wellbeing includes a sense of personal safety and security, emotional support and connection, mechanisms to cope with stressors, and access to services when appropriate for short- and long-term care. The committee believes that institutions have a responsibility both to enhance the wellbeing of all students and to provide additional support to a subset of students with more severe emotional distress and mental illness.

The Statement of Task for the Committee on Supporting the Whole Student: Mental Health, Substance Abuse, and Wellbeing in Higher Education includes the following specific tasks:

- Identify and review programs, practices, resources, and policies that institutions of higher education have developed to treat mental health issues and to support wellbeing on campuses.
- Analyze the challenges that institutions face—including financial, cultural, and human resource obstacles and methods to address these challenges.
- Investigate factors related to the funding of and access to mental health services and support for student wellbeing, such as student academic performance and campus climate.
- Examine, to the extent possible, the relationship between student mental health, wellbeing, and rates of alcohol and drug use, and recommend ways in which institutions can address substance use and its effects on campus climate.
- Produce a consensus report with recommendations, as well as derivative products that will be broadly distributed on campuses, at professional society meetings, and in other venues.

Over the course of the 18-month study, the committee held two in-person and two virtual listening sessions with university leaders and administrators, counseling center directors and staff, researchers, and students on four campuses. Participants were asked to comment on the statement of task, share related research, describe mental health services on campus (location of offices, staff organization, and description of roles), and identify issues they saw as priorities in the field. Because a significant portion of the study took place during the height of the COVID-19 outbreak, the committee's ability to meet and hold discussions in person and conduct information-gathering activities and listening sessions at institutions of various types and sizes and conferences was limited.

The committee also examined data from multiple federal agencies and national professional networks and associations and commissioned the following papers and literature reviews:

Miriam Akeju, "Behavioral Health of Students Identifying as Hispanic/ Latinx at Colleges and Universities: Existing Data, Trends, and Best Practices for Prevention, Early Intervention and Treatment."

Angie Barrall, "Substance Use Disorders: Literature Review and Research Analysis."

Nicole Braun, "Mental Illness, Substance Use, and Wellness at Community Colleges in the US: Literature Review and Research Analysis."

Susanna Harris, "A Review of Mental Health, Substance Abuse, and Well-being Resources for Students and a Review of Previous Report Recommendations in Higher Education."

David Patterson Silver Wolf; Asher Blackdeer, A.; Beeler-Stinn, S.; & Van Schuyver, J., "Behavioral Health Trends of Students Enrolled at Historically Black College and Universities and Tribal Colleges and Universities."

Finally, the committee commissioned an analysis by the Counseling Center of the University of Illinois at Urbana-Champaign of previously unpublished data on suicide rates from 2009 to 2018 at 13 campuses that are members of the Big Ten Counseling Centers, modeled on a similar study by Silverman el al., 1997. This analysis can be found in Appendix D.

In conducting its research and making its recommendations, the committee decided to craft its findings and recommendations in ways that apply across the diverse types of academic institutions, and, when possible, point out special circumstances unique to individual types of institutions. The committee also paid greater attention to educational levels and academic fields in which data on student mental health issues were available. The report, therefore, contains some information on graduate students and medical students but focuses primarily on undergraduate students. Even though the committee was asked to investigate mental health issues among Science, Technology, Engineering, Mathematics, and Medicine (STEMM) students where feasible, most of the data relevant to this study are not disaggregated by field. In any case, the issues of mental health, substance use, and wellbeing affect all students in all disciplines, as do the campus services provided to deal with them.

Although mental health issues affect students in all professional fields of study, the committee was explicitly asked by the study sponsors to focus on medical students. It has provided some information on medical students, although given the broad scope of the study, that information is necessarily brief. In its focus on medical students, the committee acknowledges that the mental health issues facing this population frequently also apply to other health professionals and students pursuing other health degrees. These mental health issues have been exacerbated by the COVID-19 crisis, where all health professionals are facing front line stresses related to the diagnosis, treatment, and care of patients and have been found to be at higher risk of developing psychological distress and other mental health symptoms.

The committee's approach was to make the majority of its recommendations suitable for all institutions and to point out exceptions to those recommendations where appropriate.

Again, the committee acknowledges that there are limited data available on the mental health of students disaggregated by field. This is unfortunate, as differences by field are likely. For example, authors of a study at California Polytechnic State University found that the university's engineering students "suffer from certain mental health issues at a much higher rate than the average U.S. college student" (Danowitz and Beddoes, 2018). Further research on fields and subfields may reveal additional information about the specific needs of that population.

DATA SOURCES AND CONSIDERATIONS

Data on mental health and substance use in students can be challenging to interpret for a number of reasons. These data are drawn from different groups of students, including those seeking mental health services in counseling centers, subjects of targeted surveys on specific problems, higher education students in general, and broader segments of an age-equivalent population in and outside academia. Also, multiple methods are used in data collection, and it is important to consider the varying strengths, limitations, and purposes of various measurement approaches.

Much of the information on the incidence of mental health and substance use problems among students is based on self-reports from general population surveys, not actual clinical evaluations. This approach has the advantage of drawing from entire student populations, regardless of contact with health services, but it is also subject to key limitations. Self-report surveys typically rely on brief screens that are correlated with but not equivalent to clinical evaluations, resulting in a certain proportion of false positives and false negatives, depending on the sensitivity and specificity of the screen. In addition, survey self-reports are vulnerable to nonresponse bias, in which systematic differences between survey respondents and nonrespondents may yield results that do not accurately represent the target population (Dang et al., 2020). At the same time, self-reported screens are an economical method for collecting data from large populations, and they remain the predominant approach to estimating the prevalence of mental health conditions in psychiatric epidemiology research.

Data from clinical settings are drawn from students who use mental health services from a counseling center in order to be evaluated or receive treatment. These data have two major strengths: the potential to characterize the full sub-population (by minimizing or eliminating nonresponse) and the ability to include assessments by clinicians instead of or in addition to self-reported symptoms. The key caveat for clinical data is that they are limited to those who use clinical services and therefore do not represent students who are not accessing those services.

No single data point, or source of data, is capable of conveying the complexity of mental health and substance use problems among students. Multiple approaches and methodologies provide contrasting angles on the same concept and contribute to a richer understanding of the issues. These different approaches need to be taken into account in forming conclusions about the prevalence of mental health and substance use issues in higher education. Chapter 6 describes some of the research needed to help address data limitations.

STRUCTURE OF THE REPORT

Recommendations in this report are directed at the various stakeholders in the U.S. postsecondary education enterprise, including federal and state policy makers and funders, institutions of higher education and their administrators and faculty, as well as the students that the system is intended to educate. The recommendations are intended to help the nation's institutions of higher education provide guidance that enables all who work and learn within it to create an environment that supports student wellbeing, establishes a culture that destigmatizes mental health issues, and provides those students in need with the appropriate services and resources. At the same time, the committee recognizes that at least some of its recommendations will require funds and institutional capacities that many community colleges, universities, and graduate and medical schools currently lack. For this reason, the committee also includes recommendations for policy makers and funders of higher education to help academic institutions bridge gaps and build capacity for long-term improvement.

As has been the case with other recent reports from the National Academies, such as *Graduate STEM Education for the 21st Century*, *The Science of Effective Mentorship in STEMM*, *Breaking Through: The Next Generation of Biomedical and Behavioral Sciences Researchers*, and *The Integration of the Humanities and Arts with Sciences, Engineering, and Medicine in Higher Education: Branches from the Same Tree*, improving student wellbeing comes down to an imperative to change institutional culture. Absent culture change, the status quo will remain. It is the committee's hope that this report will serve as a call to action to faculty members, deans, provosts, presidents, and other university administrators to address the policies and culture of the nation's institutions of higher education that adversely affect students' mental health and substance use.

Following this introductory chapter, the remainder of this report lays out the committee's analysis of the current state of students and institutions regarding mental health, substance use, and wellbeing in Chapters 2. Chapter 3 offers mental health, substance use, and wellbeing approaches, resources, and programs provided to the general student population, and Chapter 4 covers services provided to students by licensed providers or in a clinical setting. Chapter 5 examines specific challenges and barriers to change and the opportunities to address them with evidence-based interventions. Chapter 5 also contains the report's major recommendations. Chapter 6 provides a listing of major issues that require additional research if the recommendations in this report are to be fully effective once implemented.

2

Mental Health, Substance Use, and Wellbeing in Higher Education in the United States

The system of higher education in the United States is complex and diverse—both in terms of the types of degree-granting institutions and the diversity of the student populations. Both are critical considerations in framing approaches to dealing with an increasing prevalence of mental health problems and substance use within this system. This chapter begins with broad trends in higher education structures and the types of students attending them, as a foundation for the discussion of mental health trends.

THE STRUCTURE OF THE HIGHER EDUCATION SYSTEM

There are more than 4,000 institutions of higher education in the United States, both publicly and privately funded. Publicly funded institutions—most institutions of higher education—are overseen by elected or appointed boards of directors or regents. Even though similar boards oversee private institutions, both not-for-profit and for-profit, these are appointed by the institutions themselves. As a result, the individuals or entities in control of private, for-profit institutions can receive bonuses, dividends, and other financial benefits in the event of net profit. Chapter 5 provides more information about the ways in which changes come about in different types of institutions.

"Community college" is a term used in the United States to refer primarily to institutions of higher education that confer associate degrees as the terminal degree. This report will reference data related to associate degree–granting institutions, even as some community colleges have begun to offer bachelor's degrees (AACC, 2019). In 2018-2019, the approximately 1,300 community colleges in the United States served 5.7 million students or 35 percent of all undergraduate students (NCES, 2020). Community colleges are more likely to serve students who are Black, Indigenous, and people of color (BIPOC), of lower socioeconomic status, and/or are the first in their family to attend college, known as first-generation students (Snyder, de Brey, and Dillow, 2019). As of 2018, community colleges as a whole had passed the minority-majority threshold, meaning that greater than 50 percent of the students are from groups other than white. Demographic factors such as socioeconomic status, race/ethnicity, and first-generation status can increase the likelihood of academic vulnerabilities that correlate with lower rates of completion, often increasing the need for remedial coursework that community college students require at higher rates than do those at bachelor's degree–granting colleges and universities (Snyder, de Brey, and Dillow, 2019). Community colleges often have fewer resources than bachelor's degree–granting colleges and universities to serve more students who are less likely to have benefited from a strong K-12 education, safe communities, and other factors that correlate with higher socioeconomic status; thus increasing the need to make counseling and resources more available at community colleges

Under the umbrella of graduate schools, this report includes master's and doctoral degree–granting programs, as well as medical and other professional degree programs beyond the bachelor's degree. The U.S. Department of Education (ED) describes master's programs as a first-level graduate degree that takes approximately two years to complete. For research doctoral degrees (not including professional degrees), ED describes the degree as a program that includes advanced study and independent research with supervision, culminating in a dissertation or thesis. Distinct from a research doctoral degree, ED considers the Doctor of Medicine (M.D.) as a first-professional degree. In 2018-2019, there were 154 institutions that offered programs for medical education (AAMC, 2019, chart 5).

The United States also has a number of institutions that are classified as Minority Serving Institutions (MSIs), which cut across two- and four-year degree-granting institutions. MSIs traditionally fall into two categories: *historically defined* or *enrollment-defined* (see Table B-1 and Table B-2 in Appendix B).

According to the National Academies 2019 report *Minority Serving Institutions: America's Underutilized Resource for Strengthening the STEM Workforce* (NASEM, 2019a), "there are more than 700 federally designated MSIs that represent approximately 14 percent of all degree-granting, Title IV-eligible institutions of higher education. Taken together, MSIs enroll roughly five million students, or nearly 30 percent of all undergraduates in U.S. higher education" (NASEM, 2019a). MSIs as a category are themselves diverse in nature (Núñez, Hurtado, and Calderón Galeano, 2015), and there is some disagreement among different stakeholders as to how to count the number of MSIs, resulting in varying estimates of the total number of MSIs in the United States (NASEM, 2019a).

CHANGES IN STUDENT DEMOGRAPHICS

The composition of the student body at U.S. institutions of higher education has become increasingly diverse over the past decades (ACE, 2020). Colleges and universities, originally designed to serve a predominantly white and male population, have experienced a shift in the proportions of students who can be characterized by gender, race and ethnicity, socioeconomic status, citizenship, veteran status, disability status, and sexual and gender minority (SGM) status,[1] first-generation students, and students with dependents. As the representation of historically excluded groups has increased in the United States, colleges and universities have had to learn to expand their view of how to support students from different backgrounds so that the diversity of the entering classes is reflected in the diversity of those students who graduate and enter the workforce or pursue additional educational experiences (see Box 2-1 for terminology in the report).

In postsecondary education, the overall enrollment of female students achieved parity with males in the late 1970s, and the share of female students has continued to increase, reaching 57 percent of overall enrollment by 2018-2019 (Snyder, de Brey, and Dillow, 2019). There remain disciplines such as computer science, engineering, physics, and mathematics where women have been underrepresented and continue to comprise a smaller proportion of degrees conferred. Similarly, the increase in diversity in terms of race and ethnicity, both in absolute numbers and the proportion of students who are Black, Hispanic, Asian, Pacific Islander, Native Indian/Alaska Native, or of two or more races, has not translated into equal rates of graduation or fields of study (Snyder, de Brey, and Dillow, 2019).

Varying completion rates for racial and ethnic minority students suggest there are factors within higher education that fail to provide equitable support to students from BIPOC groups. It is also more likely that students from historically underrepresented racial and ethnic backgrounds come from a lower socioeconomic background and are first-generation students, two other factors that correlate with lower rates of completion (Reynolds and Cruise, 2020; Wilbur and Roscigno, 2016). Looking to future trends, the proportion of students who are Black, Hispanic, Asian, Pacific Islander, Native American/Alaska Native, and multiple-race non-Hispanic is projected to increase, and institutions of higher education will need to continue to search for opportunities to provide additional supports for these students (see Figure 2-1).

---

[1] Sexual and gender minority (SGM) populations "include, but are not limited to, individuals who identify as lesbian, gay, bisexual, asexual, transgender, Two-Spirit, queer, and/or intersex. Individuals with same-sex or -gender attractions or behaviors and those with a difference in sex development are also included. These populations also encompass those who do not self-identify with one of these terms but whose sexual orientation, gender identity or expression, or reproductive development is characterized by non-binary constructs of sexual orientation, gender, and/or sex." This definition has been provided by the Sexual & Gender Minority Research Office (SGMRO) that coordinates (SGM)-related research and activities at the National Institutes of Health.

BOX 2-1
Terms Used in This Report

For the purposes of this report, the committee will use two terms to describe groups of students: Black, Indigenous, and people of color (BIPOC) and historically excluded.

Black, Indigenous, and people of color (BIPOC): This term reflects the distinct history of discrimination, harm, and racism that the United States has caused Black and Indigenous people. The inclusion of people of color in BIPOC reflects the ways that individuals from other race and ethnic groups have also been discriminated against in the United States.

Historically Excluded: This term includes individuals who are BIPOC in addition to other identities that have had limited access to higher education and have faced broader discrimination based on gender, race and ethnicity, socioeconomic status, citizenship, sexual and gender minority status, disability, first generation student status, and their status as students with dependents. The use of "excluded" to describe the treatment of these groups represents the outcomes of policies used to discriminate against these people with these identities whether or not they were developed intentionally. Thus, this term includes discrimination caused to individuals from these groups from implicit bias and unintended policies. The use of exclusion is meant to capture the impact of the actions rather than the intent, as the individuals in these groups experienced reduced access to higher education and a less welcoming environment.

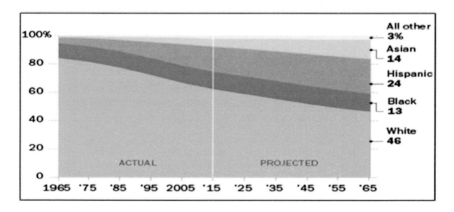

FIGURE 2-1 Changing U.S. demographics from 1965 to 2065, percentage of the total population.
Note: Whites, Blacks, and Asians include only single-race non-Hispanics; Asians include Pacific Islanders. Other races include Native American/Alaska Native and multiple-race non-Hispanics. Hispanics can be of any race.
Source: Taylor, 2016.

The data above reflect gender as a category and race and ethnic background as a separate category; however, the tendency to disaggregate and present data by these dimensions alone does not reflect the fact that people live with overlapping identities and belong to many groups. The term "intersectionality" refers to the multiple identities that students hold and how those identities interact. The term intersectionality was originally coined by legal scholar Kimberlé Crenshaw to describe the combined experience of Black women facing both sexism and racism, but has been broadened to describe "the interconnected nature of social categorizations such as race, class, and gender, regarded as creating overlapping and interdependent systems of discrimination or disadvantage" (Crenshaw, 1989; McCall, 2005).

This report also examines other groups of interest to higher education, including, but not limited to, students with disabilities, students from lower socioeconomic status, first-generation students, veterans, student-athletes, and students who are SGM students. Many of these students often fall into the category of what the Postsecondary National Policy Institute (PNPI) calls the "post-traditional student." According to PNPI, nearly 15 percent of the U.S. undergraduate population would be considered "traditional" students, i.e., those between 17 and 21 years old who attend 4-year colleges and live on campus (PNPI, 2020b). The remaining 85 percent of students enrolled in the nation's colleges and universities include adult learners, working parents, full-time workers, low-income students, and students who commute to school.

Some demographic groups and identities intersect more often than others do. For example, student veterans are more likely to be older, have dependents, and have a higher rate of reporting disability than non-veteran students (26 percent versus 19 percent) (NCES, 2019). As will be described later in this chapter, students who are BIPOC are also more likely to be first-generation students and to come from lower socioeconomic status. An intersectional understanding of student identities is a way to see the cumulative impact of discriminatory policies, unequal distribution of wealth across demographic groups, and other systemic inequities that have caused harm. Colleges and universities seeking to create equitable representation in enrollment across all groups must recognize the ways that the legacy of these historical practices fail to serve the many dimensions of the students who seek degrees today.

TRENDS IN MENTAL HEALTH AND SUBSTANCE USE IN HIGHER EDUCATION

Over the past two decades, numerous reports from higher education stakeholders have drawn attention to the increasingly complex concerns relating to mental health among students in postsecondary education (Duffy et al., 2019, 2020). The media, as well as some leaders in higher education, has categorized the current situation as a crisis—citing the facts that more students than ever report symptoms consistent with mental illness, that substance use continues to be a serious problem on campuses, and that there has been a dramatic increase in students' being referred to and utilizing mental health services. The COVID-19 pandemic has exacerbated the situation. It is negatively impacting students, as it is the entire population, in ways we do not yet fully understand. Some recent studies have identified examples of that impact at specific institutions; in one study, students reported more stress and anxiety due to the COVID-19 outbreak (Son et al., 2020), and in another, researchers found that, compared with prior academic terms, students who were enrolled during COVID-19, "were more sedentary, anxious, and depressed" (Huckins et al., 2020). How those impacts compare with increases in anxiety and stress in the general population is unknown.

However, the current situation, including the long-term impact of the pandemic, is difficult to assess accurately and quite complex. As one group of researchers has argued, "[...] based on this evidence, it is tempting to conclude that more college students in recent years are suffering from mood disorders. However, increases in service utilization could be caused by many factors other than increased prevalence, including greater awareness, better accessibility of services, improved outreach, or other factors not rooted in a true increase in prevalence" (Duffy, Twenge, and Joiner, 2019).

In addition, over the past 15 years numerous federal, state, and private funding mechanisms, including the Garret Lee Smith Memorial Act, have invested hundreds of millions of dollars toward reducing stigma, increasing help-seeking, and training gate-keepers; all of which lead to increased rates of identification and referral of students for treatment. Whether or not the state of mental health in higher education constituted a crisis, the simultaneous triad of COVID-19, the economic downturn, and long-standing racism and racial oppression did not improve the general living conditions of those living and receiving education in the United States.

Thus, institutions of higher education face the challenge of meeting a broad range of students' needs in the context of increasing distress and demand for services at the same moment in time when leadership must make decisions about virtual or in-person enrollment, pandemic protocols, and even more uncertain budgets. These challenges come at a time when higher education has received the greatest decline in public financial support in decades, resulting in tight budgets and difficult allocation decisions. In terms of mental health, colleges and universities are also operating in the larger U.S. context of unequally distributed therapeutic, psychological, and psychiatric services across the nation. Access to these services may be reduced as a result of the cost of health insurance, limited coverage of mental health services by insurance companies, the number of private providers who accept insurance or referrals for a given insurance type, and the concentration of providers in any given area. The challenges for colleges and universities, aligned with the state of U.S. mental health services generally, serves as the context for the following trends.

National Data Sources and Considerations

While the overall trends presented in the sections above provide a starting point for understanding the trends in mental health and substance use in higher education, the existing data do not provide a thorough understanding of all populations in higher education. Articles on college and university mental health, for example, often cite age-matched data. These data are useful for understanding context and broader mental health trends in young adults as a whole, but they may not necessarily reflect the prevalence of mental health issues in students. For example, having national data that can be disaggregated between students enrolled in higher education and those who are not would allow researchers to make comparisons between college and age-matched peers (see Box 2-2).

The degree to which existing datasets can be disaggregated by gender, race and ethnic group, nationality, veteran status, SGM status, first-generation student status, socioeconomic status, and other characteristics varies. As colleges and universities address discrimination and bias in admissions, campus leaders, researchers, and public health providers would benefit from understanding national trends for these groups, as well as for those at their own institution (see Chapter 3). Going forward, it would be helpful to collect information that could be disaggregated by types of institutions and programs, notably community colleges, MSIs, graduate programs, and programs that enroll students primarily in hybrid or online models. Community colleges and MSIs, which serve more students who are BIPOC and first-generation students, often have fewer financial resources to collect data. A better understanding of their circumstances could help those campuses make more effective decisions in terms of programs and avenues for support (see Box 2-3).

An additional data issue arises from the fact that general population estimates are affected by survey nonresponse. Students who participate in the surveys could be systematically different from those who do not (e.g., more attuned to or interested in mental health concerns), which could bias the estimates upwards or downwards relative to the true population values. Similarly, screening instruments used in general population surveys, such as the nine-item major depression module of the Patient Health Questionnaire (PHQ-9), are known to significantly overestimate prevalence rates (Levis et al., 2020). The useful and oft-cited Healthy Minds Study, for example, uses survey sample weights based on known characteristics of the full population (e.g., gender, race/ethnicity, academic level, and grade point average distribution), but a follow-up study indicated that initial survey participants were more likely than nonrespondents to have symptoms of depression and use mental health services (Eisenberg, Golberstein, and Gollust, 2007). Additional discussion of self-reported data from general population surveys compared to data from clinical diagnoses can be found in Chapter 1.

BOX 2-2
National Data Sources of Mental Health,
Substance Use, and Wellbeing

There are key differences in the types of national data available to illustrate the trends in mental health, substance use, and wellbeing in higher education. Some databases provide data drawn from college students receiving mental health services. These data, such as those collected by the Center for Collegiate Mental Health (CCMH), represent the population of students seeking services across the nation as well as data provided by the clinicians who treat them. Clinical data are drawn from students who have sought care from their college or university counseling center, however, and not all students seek care or have access to care. In contrast, general population surveys—another important data source—provide information based on individual self-reported symptoms that represent a measure of symptom prevalence in the population that is generalized from students who respond to the surveys. These two types of data are important information that can be considered in parallel, and this report will reference both clinical and general population data to identify trends. Below is a list of national data sources for mental health, substance use, and wellbeing in higher education and for young adults.

Center for Collegiate Mental Health at Pennsylvania State University: CCMH started in 2004, is a Practice-Research-Network dedicated to the field of college student mental health. CCMH brings science and practice together by collecting aggregate, de-identified, standardized mental health data through routine clinical practice from more than 650 college counseling center members. CCMH manages a variety of standardized data points, including the Counseling Center Assessment of Psychological Symptoms (CCAPS), a multi-dimensional assessment instrument, most recently updated in 2019, with norms based on 448,904 students seeking counseling services. The CCAPS is available in multiple lengths, used for both intake and routine outcome monitoring, and includes eight subscales: Depression, Generalized Anxiety, Social Anxiety, Academic Distress, Eating Concerns, Family Distress, Hostility, Substance Use, and a generalized Distress Index. CCMH also developed the Standardized Data Set (SDS), a standardized set of questions typically used at intake to collect demographic information about clients receiving mental health treatment at college counseling centers. Currently, CCMH has a data set of 998,013 unique students served in counseling centers from 2010 to 2020. Other information is drawn from appointment types and information provided by clinicians during treatment.

Healthy Minds Survey (HMS) at the University of Michigan, University of California, Los Angeles, and Boston University: HMS is an annual web-based general population survey study examining mental health, service utilization, and related issues among undergraduate and graduate students. Since its national launch in 2007, HMS has been fielded at about 300 colleges and universities, with more than 300,000 survey respondents. HMS is one of the only annual surveys of college and university populations that focuses exclusively on mental health and related issues, allowing for substantial detail in this area. The study has a special emphasis on understanding service utilization and help-seeking behavior, including factors such as stigma, knowledge, and the role of peers and other potential gatekeepers.

Monitoring the Future Survey administered by the National Institute on Drug Abuse and the University of Michigan: Since 1975 the Monitoring the Future (MTF) general population survey has measured drug and alcohol use and related attitudes among adolescent students nationwide. Survey participants report their drug use behaviors across three time periods: lifetime, past-year, and past-month. Overall, 42,531 students from 396 public and private schools participated in this year's MTF survey. The survey is funded by the National Institute on Drug Abuse (NIDA), a component of the National Institutes of Health (NIH), and conducted by the University of Michigan.

National College Health Assessment from the American College Health Association (ACHA): The ACHA-National College Health Assessment II (ACHA-NCHA II) is a national, general population research study organized by ACHA to assist college health service providers, health educators, counselors, and administrators in collecting data about their students' habits, behaviors, and perceptions on the most prevalent health topics. ACHA initiated the original ACHA-NCHA in 2000, and the instrument was used nationwide through the spring 2008 data collection period. The ACHA-NCHA now provides the largest known comprehensive data set on the health of college students, providing the college health and higher education fields with a vast spectrum of information on student health. The survey has undergone two revisions, the ACHA-NCHA II from 2008 to 2018 and the ACHA-NCHA III starting in fall 2019. For consistency across time periods, this report uses the ACHA-NCAHA II. For the fall 2018 survey, there were 40 institutions, 26,181 students, a mean response proportion of 17 percent, and a median response proportion of 12 percent.

National Survey of Drug Use and Health (NSDUH) administered by the Substance Abuse and Mental Health Services Administration: NSDUH is representative of persons aged 12 and over in the civilian noninstitutionalized population of the United States, and in each state and the District of Columbia. The general population survey covers residents of households (including those living in houses, townhouses, apartments, and condominiums), persons in non-institutional group quarters (including those in shelters, boarding houses, college dormitories, migratory work camps, and halfway houses), and civilians living on military bases. People excluded from the survey include those experiencing homelessness who do not use shelters, active military personnel, and residents of institutional group quarters such as jails, nursing homes, mental institutions, and long-term care hospitals. While this is not specific to higher education, the survey data include indicators for age-match comparisons to enrolled students.

BOX 2-3
Data Collection at Tribal Colleges and Universities and
Limited Data on Indigenous and Native American Students

Compared to other types of institutions, there is a notable data shortage for Tribal Colleges and Universities (TCUs). The National Student Clearinghouse (NSC) reports that 84 percent of Title IV degree-granting institutions—those that process U.S. federal student aid and whose students, if demonstrating financial need, can receive student loans and grants and enter a work-study program—report their data to the clearinghouse (Dundar and Shapiro, 2016), compared to only 35 percent of TCUs (Espinosa, Turk, and Taylor, 2018). While one solution to this data issue would be to have more of the 34 TCUs reporting into the clearinghouse or other data collections, there are a number of internal, external, and historical factors that create significant challenges to realizing that solution. Understanding and addressing these factors, then, has to be the first step before it will be possible to resolve the data issue for TCUs (Espinosa, Turk, and Taylor, 2018).

The tribal college movement began in the 1960s and 1970s to address the problem that Native and Indigenous students were not persisting and graduating from predominantly white colleges and universities. Advocates of establishing tribal colleges saw these institutions as a way to build the intellectual capacity that best served individual tribal nations and their students (McSwain and Cunningham, 2006). Today, 32 TCUs enroll nearly 28,000 full- and part-time students annually. Between 2002 and 2012, overall enrollment at TCUs increased by 9 percent (Espinosa, Turk, and Taylor, 2018).

One issue for TCUs is that NSC and other large data warehouses do not employ measures, frame data collection, and report the types of data that can

TRENDS IN MENTAL HEALTH IN HIGHER EDUCATION

In the sections that follow regarding trends in mental health, it is important to understand how trend data are interpreted. In addition to the differences mentioned previously between self-reported data and clinical data, there is also variation in the types of instruments used for screens and diagnostics that can yield significantly different results. For this reason, some of the figures associated with each trend include data points from multiple sources with notations on the instrument used to create a more nuanced understanding of the trend. Figures with multiple data sets include data from the 2013-14 and 2018-19 academic years.

Trends in Student Anxiety

According to the National Institute of Mental Health (NIMH), people with generalized anxiety disorder (GAD) "display excessive anxiety or worry, most days for at least six months, about a number of things such as personal health, capture the effects that TCUs are making at the community level, such as engaging in coursework and outreach to save and revitalize tribal language and culture. Often, TCUs create curricula and community events to share tribal knowledge with all community members, even those not enrolled in college (Espinosa, Turk, and Taylor, 2018).

TCUs have collaborated with tribally informed organizations, such as the American Indian Higher Education Consortium (AIHEC) and the American Indian College Fund (the College Fund), to begin reporting data relevant to TCUs and their communities and to collect data on mental health and substance use among students at TCUs. For example, through a partnership between the University of Washington's Indigenous Wellness Research Institute (IWRI) Northwest Indian College, AIHEC, and advocates at several additional TCUs, a team at IWRI used a community-based participatory research approach that "engages tribal community constituents in decision-making and power-sharing in all aspects of the process, including planning, implementation, analysis, ownership of data, and dissemination of results" to gain a better understanding of alcohol and drug use at TCUs. With funding from the National Institutes of Drug Abuse and approval from 27 TCUs, the team carried out a web-based survey to understand TCU community members' perceptions of problems with underage drinking and drug use, as well as to identify promising practices for addressing these issues on TCU campuses. Outside of TCUs, data on Native American and Indigenous students are also scarce. Often, these students appear as an "asterisked" group in data because of statistical insignificance (Espinosa, Turk, and Taylor, 2018). Given the limited data on educational outcomes for Native American and Indigenous students, generalizations about BIPOC students as a group do not reflect the issues relevant to these students (see Chapter 6 for additional recommendations in the research agenda in terms of supporting data collection).

work, social interactions, and everyday routine life circumstances. The fear and anxiety can cause significant problems in areas of their life" (NIMH, 2020a). Symptoms may include restlessness, fatigue, difficulty concentrating, irritability, muscle tension, intrusive feelings of worry, and sleep problems.

Data from HMS[2] show there has been an increase in the percentage of students self-reporting symptoms of generalized anxiety (based on the GAD-7

---

[2] Each participating school provides the Health Minds Study team with a randomly selected sample of currently enrolled students over the age of 18. Large schools typically provide a random sample of 4,000 students, while smaller schools typically provide a sample of all students. Schools with graduate students typically include both undergraduates and graduate students in the sample. The overall participation rate for the 2018-2019 study was 16 percent. It is important to raise the question of whether the 16 percent who participated are different in important ways from the 84 percent who did not participate. We address this issue by constructing nonresponse weights using administrative data on full student populations. Most of the 79 schools in the 2018-2019 HMS were able to provide administrative data about all randomly selected students.

screen) from 17.2 percent with a positive screen (GAD-7 ≥10) in 2013 to 31.2 percent in 2019.[3] There has also been an increase in students screening positive for severe anxiety (GAD-7 ≥15) from 6 percent in 2013 to 13.5 percent in 2018 (see Table 2-1).

Over the 2007-2019 time period, 30.7 percent of female students reported anxiety in comparison to 19.7 percent of male students. There are also differences over the same time period by race and ethnic group (see Figure 2-2).

There are other more generalized ways that surveys have captured the sense of anxiety from students. NCHA includes the following question to the undergraduate participants, who self-report their symptoms: "Have you ever felt

TABLE 2-1 Comparison of Measures of Anxiety in Higher Education Students from Multiple Sources in 2013 and 2018

	Year		
Measures of Anxiety	Fall 2013	Fall 2018	% Change 2013-2018
CCMH: CAPPS-34 Subscale scores for generalized anxiety[a]	1.86	2.03	9.1
CCMH: CAPPS-34 Subscale scores social anxiety[a]	1.87	2.03	8.6
HMS: Percentage of students self-reporting anxiety (based on the GAD-7 ≥10 screen)[b]	17.2%	31.3%	81.9
HMS: Percent of students self-reporting severe anxiety (GAD-7 ≥15 Screen)[b]	6.0%	13.5%	125.0
ACHA-NCHA: Have you ever felt overwhelming anxiety anytime within the last 12 months?[c]	51.0%	62.3%	22.2
NCHA: Have you felt overwhelming anger in the last 12 months?[c]	35.6%	41.7%	17.1
NCHA: Within the last 12 months, have you been diagnosed or treated by a professional for anxiety?[c]	8.0%	22.0%	175.0

[a]CCMH (clinical data); [b]HMS (general population data); [c]NCHA (general population data)
Sources: ACHA, 2014, 2018; CCMH, 2015, 2020b; HMN, 2020.

---

[3] Using the GAD 7-item scale. Each participating school provides the HMS team with a randomly selected sample of currently enrolled students over the age of 18. Large schools typically provide a random sample of 4,000 students, while smaller schools typically provide a sample of all students. Schools with graduate students typically include both undergraduates and graduate students in the sample. Undergraduate students include community college students.

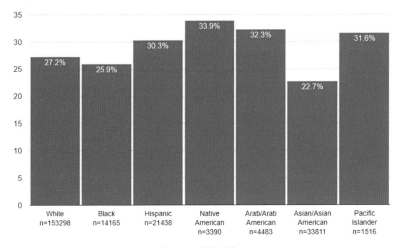

Race and Ethnicity

FIGURE 2-2 Percentage of student self-reported screens of anxiety by race, 2007-2019. Source: Healthy Minds Network.

overwhelming anxiety?"[4] In the 2011-2012 the response was 51.1 percent compared to 63.6 in 2017-2018. While not the same as anxiety, the study reports that 37.7 percent of students felt overwhelming anger in 2011-2012 and 42.9 percent in 2017-2018 (Duffy, Twenge, and Joiner, 2019). On the other hand, clinical data provided by CCMH suggest smaller increases in average levels of student-self-reported generalized and social anxiety from 2013 to 2018 (9.1 percent and 8.6 percent, respectively), alongside massive increases in the number of students being treated in college counseling centers.

---

[4] Response options for all items were "No, never," "No, not in the last 12 months," "Yes, in the last 2 weeks," "Yes, in the last 30 days," and "Yes, in the last 12 months." For analyses, frequencies of each item endorsed within the last 2 weeks, 30 days, or 12 months were summed to produce an incidence value for 12-month prevalence for each semester. These were then weighted and summed within academic years, resulting in one value per academic year for each item. The wording of these items and their administration did not differ during the assessed years.

Participants were 610,543 undergraduate U.S. college students who participated in the American College Health Association's NCHA between fall 2011 and spring 2018. The NCHA is a large, national survey of college health administered each semester. Participating universities recruited random samples of enrolled students to complete either paper or web-based surveys of past-year beliefs and behaviors regarding a variety of health and health-risk variables. Participants are required to be aged 18 years or older. Participation is voluntary, and response rates averaged 22 percent from 2011 to 2018. Data for the current project were drawn from biannual Undergraduate Reference Group Reports made publicly available online by the American College Health Association for the 2011-2012 to 2017-2018 academic years (available at https://www.acha.org/NCHA/ACHA-NCHA_Data/Publications_and_Reports/NCHA/Data/Publications_and_Reports.aspx?hkey=d5fb767c-d15d-4efc-8c41-3546d92032c5 [accessed October 1, 2020].

Trends in Depression

Depression is a common and serious mood disorder that can affect how the individual feels, thinks, and manages daily activities with inhibitions and limitations lasting for two weeks or more. The presentation of depression varies, and it may develop in specific situations, including during specific seasons or after giving birth. Major symptoms can include feeling sad or angry, hopeless, worthless, or irritable; decreased energy; loss of interest in previously enjoyed activities; difficulty with concentration or memory recall; difficulty sleeping; changes in weight; thoughts of death or self-harm; and physical ailments that do not have a clear connection to another physical cause (NIMH, 2020e).

The Healthy Minds Network study reported an increase in positive screens for depression (PHQ09 score ≥10) from 22 percent of students in 2007 to 36.4 percent in 2019.[5] There has also been an increase in the rate of students self-reporting symptoms of major depression (PHQ-9 ≥15), from 8.8 percent in 2013 to 18 percent in 2019 (see Table 2-2).[6]

Over the same timeframe, more women (31.5 percent) reported symptoms consistent with any level of depression than men (24.8 percent). There are also differences in depression rates by race and ethnicity, with Native American students reporting the highest level of depression (38.7 percent) (see Figure 2-3); by citizenship, with more U.S. citizens reporting having depression (29.5 percent) than international students (25.9 percent); and by degree level, with 31.3 percent of undergraduates, 21.1 percent of master's degree students, and 21.1 percent of students pursuing other degrees (HMN, 2007-2019).

NCHA provides another data point for depression in undergraduates, with the survey asking students to self-report to the question, "Have you ever felt so depressed that it was difficult to function?" For this data set, participants responded at 31.5 percent in 2011-12 and 42.2 percent in 2017-18 (Duffy, Twenge, and Joiner, 2019). Over the same period of time, and again in contrast to nonclinical population surveys, clinical data from CCMH indicated a dramatically smaller increase (6.7 percent) in self-reported levels of depression among college students seeking counseling, despite increases in the numbers of students in treatment.

---

[5] Using the Patient Health Questionnaire (PHQ), a nine-item instrument based on the symptoms provided in the *Diagnostic and Statistical Manual for Mental Disorders* for a major depressive episode in the past two weeks (Spitzer, Kroenke, and Williams, 1999). Following the standard algorithm for interpreting the PHQ-9, symptom levels are categorized as severe (score of 15+), moderate (score of 10-14), or mild/minimal (score <10).

[6] Some studies suggest that the PHQ overestimates diagnoses of depression: "The PHQ-9 is often used to generate what are described by researchers as depression prevalence estimates. The present study found that using PHQ-9 ≥10 to assess depression prevalence, which is commonly done, overestimated depression prevalence compared with prevalence based on actual diagnostic criteria by 11.9 percent (mean ratio: 2.5 times)" (Levis et al., 2020).

TABLE 2-2 Comparison of Measures of Depression in Higher Education Students from Multiple Sources in 2013 and 2018

	Year		
Measures of Depression	Fall 2013	Fall 2018	% Change 2013-2018
CCMH: CAPS-34 Subscale scores for depression[a]	1.63	1.74	6.7
HMS: Percentage of students self-reporting positive screens for any depression (PHQ-9 Score Screening ≥10) [b]	22.3%	37.1%	66.4
HMS: Percent of students self-reporting major depression (PHQ-9 Score Screening ≥15)[b]	8.8%	18.4%	109.0
NCHA: Have you felt very sad within the last 12 months? [c]	59.5%	67.9%	14.6
NCHA: Have you felt so depressed that it was difficult to function in the last 12 months?[c]	30.9%	41.4%	34.0
NCHA: Within the last 12 months, have you been diagnosed or treated by a professional for depression?[c]	7.5%	17.3%	130.7

[a]CCMH (clinical data); [b]HMS (general population data); [c]NCHA (general population data)
Sources: ACHA, 2014, 2018; CCMH, 2015, 2020b; HMN, 2007-2019.

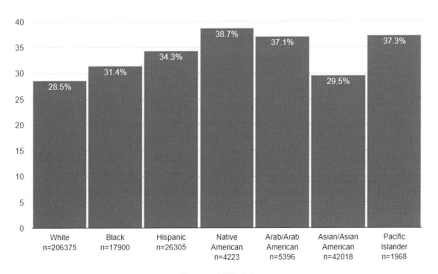

FIGURE 2-3 Percentage of student self-reported screens of depression by race, 2007-2019.
Source: Healthy Minds Network.

Trends in Other Mental Disorders

While the number of students being treated or self-reporting diagnoses for the mental disorders described may be smaller than for anxiety and depression, they remain important considerations for institutions of higher education. Anorexia nervosa, attention-deficit/hyperactivity disorder, autism spectrum disorder, bipolar disorder, bulimia nervosa, obsessive-compulsive disorder (OCD), and schizophrenia all appear on the ACHA's annual National College Health Survey.[7]

- **Anorexia nervosa**: "People with anorexia nervosa may see themselves as overweight, even when they are dangerously underweight. People with anorexia nervosa typically weigh themselves repeatedly, severely restrict the amount of food they eat, often exercise excessively, and/or may force themselves to vomit or use laxatives to lose weight. Anorexia nervosa has the highest mortality rate of any mental disorder. While many people with this disorder die from complications associated with starvation, others die of suicide" (NIMH, 2020f).

- **Attention-deficit/hyperactivity disorder (ADHD)**: "ADHD is a disorder that makes it difficult for a person to pay attention and control impulsive behaviors. He or she may also be restless and almost constantly active…Although the symptoms of ADHD begin in childhood, ADHD can continue through adolescence and adulthood. Even though hyperactivity tends to improve as a child becomes a teen, problems with inattention, disorganization, and poor impulse control often continue through the teen years and into adulthood" (NIMH, 2020b).

- **Autism spectrum disorder (ASD)**: "ASD is a developmental disorder that affects communication, behavior, and the ability to function in school, work, or other areas of life. Although ASD can be diagnosed at any age, symptoms generally appear in the first two years of life" (NIMH, 2020c).

- **Bipolar disorder** "(formerly called manic-depressive illness or manic depression) is a mental disorder that causes unusual shifts in mood, energy, activity levels, concentration, and the ability to carry out day-to-day tasks. There are three types of bipolar disorder. All three types involve clear

---

[7] 134 postsecondary institutions self-selected to participate in the Spring 2019 ACHA National College Health Assessment (ACHA, 2019b), and 86,851 surveys were completed by students on these campuses. For the purpose of forming the Reference Group, only institutions located in the United States that surveyed all students or used a random sampling technique are included in the analysis, yielding a final data set consisting of 67,972 students at 98 schools. Demographic characteristics of the 98 campuses including public, private, two-year and four-year institutions, as well as associate through doctoral programs.

changes in mood, energy, and activity levels. These moods range from periods of extremely 'up,' elated, irritable, or energized behavior (known as manic episodes) to very 'down,' sad, indifferent, or hopeless periods (known as depressive episodes). Less severe manic periods are known as hypomanic episodes" (NIMH, 2020d).

- **Bulimia nervosa:** "People with bulimia nervosa have recurrent and frequent episodes of eating unusually large amounts of food and feeling a lack of control over these episodes. This binge-eating is followed by behavior that compensates for the overeating such as forced vomiting, excessive use of laxatives or diuretics, fasting, excessive exercise, or a combination of these behaviors. People with bulimia nervosa may be slightly underweight, normal weight, or overweight" (NIMH, 2020f).

- **Obsessive-compulsive disorder (OCD)** "is a common, chronic, and long-lasting disorder in which a person has uncontrollable, reoccurring thoughts (obsessions) and/or behaviors (compulsions) that he or she feels the urge to repeat over and over" (NIMH, 2020i).

- **Schizophrenia** "is a chronic and severe mental disorder that affects how a person thinks, feels, and behaves. People with schizophrenia may seem like they have lost touch with reality. Although schizophrenia is not as common as other mental disorders, the symptoms can be very disabling" (NIMH, 2020j).

These conditions, some of which are chronic, may require more specialized treatment beyond the scope of a campus counseling center. Students report having a diagnosis or treatment for each of these disorders within the past 12 months at higher rates in both genders in 2018 than 2008, with the exception of bulimia in female students with remained flat at 1.4 percent.

For ADHD, the use of drugs such as Ritalin and Adderall in children since the early 1990s has changed management and treatment. These drugs were developed to help support learning and focus in students, garnering widespread use over the decade (Advokat and Scheithauer, 2013; Scheffler et al., 2007). The Centers for Disease Control and Prevention (CDC) reported in 2016 that some 6.1 million (9.4 percent) of children between ages 2-17 years had a diagnosis of ADHD, up from 4.4 million in 2003. Over time, more individuals who received diagnoses of ADHD and began treatment at a young age have graduated from secondary education, and many have entered postsecondary education. Increased awareness of and treatment for ADHD have raised the number of students with mental illness who may not have been able to complete a postsecondary education previously;

however, the change in the student population may not have been met by the appropriate changes in resources or support for those students.

Trends in Self-Harm, Suicidal Ideation, and Suicidality

The National Alliance on Mental Illness describes non-suicidal self-injury or self-harm as act where an individual hurts themselves on purpose. This act, which can present as cutting, burning, pulling out hair, or picking at wounds, is considered a sign of emotional distress (NAMI, 2020). NCHA, which contains data related to undergraduate students, shows an increase in the self-reporting to the question "Have you ever intentionally cut, burned, bruised, or otherwise injured yourself?" from 5.9 percent in 2012-2013 to 8.5 percent in 2017-2018 (see Table 2-3). In addition to intentional self-harm, public health officials list suicide and associated behavior as a major concern:

- **Suicide** is defined as death caused by self-directed injurious behavior with intent to die as a result of the behavior.
- A **suicide attempt** is a non-fatal, self-directed, potentially injurious behavior with intent to die as a result of the behavior. A suicide attempt might not result in injury.
- **Suicidal ideation** refers to thinking about, considering, or planning suicide (NIMH, 2020k).

The Healthy Minds Network reports an increase in students reporting non-suicidal self-injury in the past year from 14.3 percent in 2007 to 23.8 percent in 2019. Women had a higher rate of non-suicidal self-injury in the past year (20.8 percent) than men (17.4 percent), and U.S. citizens and permanent residents had a higher rate than international students (20.4 percent compared to 16 percent, respectively). Undergraduate students had a higher rate (21.9 percent) than master's students (12.1 percent). There are differences in rates reported across racial and ethnic groups, as shown in Figure 2-4.

From the NCHA, the responses from undergraduate students to the question "Have you ever seriously considered suicide" rose from 7.4 percent in 2011-2012 to 13.0 percent in 2017-2018. There have been increases in self-reported suicidal ideation over the previous 12 months from 6 percent of students in 2007 to 14.1 percent in 2019. According to data from HMS, the proportion of students reporting having a plan of suicide within the past year also increased from 1.5 percent in 2007 to 6.3 percent in 2019, while attempts to die by suicide rose from 0.6 percent in 2007 to 1.5 percent in 2019. Women reported a slightly higher rate of suicidal ideation (10.7 percent) than men (9.7 percent), as did U.S. students (11.0 percent) compared to international students (7.5 percent); and undergraduate students compared to master's students and those pursuing other degrees (11.7

TABLE 2-3 Comparison of Measures of Self-Harm, Suicidal Ideation, and Death by Suicide in Higher Education Students from Multiple Sources in 2013 and 2018

Measures of Self-Harm, Suicidal Ideation, and Death by Suicide	Fall 2013 (%)	Fall 2018 (%)	Change 2013-2018 (%)
CCMH: Percentage of students reporting a non-suicidal self-injury (lifetime) [a]	23.8	28.7	20.6
CCMH: Serious suicidal ideation (lifetime) [b]	30.9	36.7	18.8
CCMH: Suicide attempts (lifetime) [a]	8.9	10.6	21.3
HMS: Non-suicidal self-injury within last year [b]	16.7	23.8	42.5
HMS: Suicidal ideation within last year [b]	8.3	13.4	61.4
HMS: Suicide plan within last year [b]	2.4	5.8	141.7
HMS: Suicide attempt within last year [b]	0.6	1.5	150.0
NCHA: Have you intentionally cut, burned, bruised, or otherwise hurt yourself in the last 12 months? [c]	5.9	7.4	25.4
NCHA: Have you seriously considered suicide in the last 12 months? [c]	7.5	11.3	50.7
NCHA: Have you attempted suicide in the last 12 months? [c]	1.4	1.9	35.7

[a]CCMH (clinical data); [b]HMS (general population data); [c]NCHA (general population data)
Sources: ACHA, 2014, 2018; CCMH, 2015, 2020b; HMN, 2007-2019.

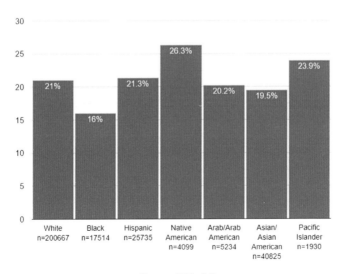

Race and Ethnicity

FIGURE 2-4 Student self-reported non-suicidal self-injury within 12 months by race, 2007-2019. Source: Healthy Minds Network.

percent vs. 6.3 percent vs. 6.8 percent, respectively). A breakdown by race and ethnicity is provided in Figure 2-5.

During the same period, clinical data related to self-harm and suicidality reported by CCMH illustrated variable rates of change in comparison to non-clinical data from HMS and NCHA. These differential rates and trends raise important questions related to determining prevalence rates. For example, in 2018 CCMH reported that 28.7 percent of students reported *lifetime* prevalence of self-harm within the population of students seeking mental health services whereas HMS reported that 23.8 percent of those responding to a general population survey reported self-injuring *in* [just] *the last year.* The similarity of these data points for such different populations across such different time periods highlights the challenges associated with accurately measuring prevalence rates for difficult-to-assess concerns such as suicidal ideation. Further underscoring this challenge, clinical data provided by CCMH in 2018 indicated that 39.6 percent of students seeking treatment reported "thoughts of ending my life" (in the last two weeks) (0< on a scale of 0 to 4) in comparison to 8.2 percent of students "seriously considered attempting suicide" (in the last month). Moreover, following a clinical assessment, clinicians identified suicidality as a presenting concern for 9.9 percent of students seeking services. Thus, even within population-level clinical data, it

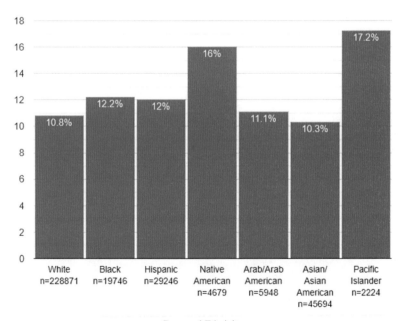

FIGURE 2-5 Percentage of student self-reported suicidal ideation by race, 2007-2019. Source: Healthy Minds Network.

appears that students may endorse different items in dramatically different ways and that professional assessment of student distress, when compared to student self-report, may produce dramatically different results. Examples such as this, viewed alongside the known tendency for screening instruments used in general population surveys, to overestimate prevalence rates, should encourage caution when interpreting data points as evidence of prevalence.

A comparison of students enrolled full-time with those of similar age (18-22) not attending college indicates that enrollment in higher education may offer a small protective factor against suicidal ideation, plans, and attempts. For example, up to 7.7 percent of full-time undergraduate and graduate students reported seriously considering suicide as compared to 9 percent of those people not enrolled in higher education (ACHA, 2012; SAMHSA and NSDUH, 2014). Similarly, up to 1.2 percent of enrolled students reported attempting suicide as compared with 2.2 percent of their age-matched peers not enrolled in college (ACHA, 2012).

In terms of demographics, there are correlations that are worth noting given the importance of the issues related to self-harm and death by suicide. In the general population men die by suicide more than women, although women engage in self-harm and related behaviors more frequently than men. Non-Hispanic white students (Nock et al., 2008) and non-heterosexual students (Figueiredo and Abreu, 2015) have a higher risk of engaging in suicidal behavior, and while the extent to which culture and identity predict suicidal behavior in college and university students is unknown, students with disabilities tend to have more suicidal ideation than students without disabilities (Coduti et al., 2016). Research has found that students who seek psychotherapy are more depressed, hostile, and anxious than students who do not seek such help, and they are three times more likely to report high levels of suicide ideation and five times more likely to have made a previous suicide attempt (Hayes et al., 2020; McAleavey et al., 2012). These latter findings also highlight questions about why rates in the general population appear to be rising so much faster than rates in the clinical populations.

Research has also identified protective factors that can lower the risk of suicidal behavior in the general public. For college students, in addition to being enrolled in higher education, research has found that not living alone is a protective factor (Hayes et al., 2020).

While there have been great attention and concern raised in recent decades in media following student death by suicide, formally identifying the annual number of deaths per year is difficult to ascertain. There is no national database, registry, or single study that collects data on death by suicide. In addition, student deaths by suicide that occur during breaks, in off-campus housing, or when a student has taken medical leave to address health concerns may not be counted consistently. CDC notes that the rates for death by suicide for age-matched individuals ages 20-24 increased 36 percent from 12.5 deaths per 100,000 in 2000 to 17.0 deaths per 100,000 in 2017, with a greater rate of increase from 2013 to 2017 (6 percent annually, on average) than from 2000 to 2013 (1 percent annually) (Curtin and

Heron, 2019). As of 2018, for age groups 15-24 and 24-35, suicide was the second highest cause of death after unintentional injury (CDC, 2019).

An important source of information on student deaths on college campuses is the ongoing study of suicides at 13 Big Ten university campuses conducted by the Big Ten Counseling Centers, based on a comprehensive 10-year study by Silverman et al. in 1997. A follow-up study of student deaths by suicide from 2009 to 2018 on these campuses was commissioned for this report. It is described in Box 2-4 (below) and included as Appendix D.

The information in Box 2-4 should not be taken as representative of the breadth of the scope of this report, as it only includes the institutions in the Big Ten Counseling Centers. These colleges and universities are large, research-oriented institutions that include undergraduate and graduate students. The Big Ten Counseling Centers does not include any community colleges or minority serving institutions.

Despite this caution, this study is actually quite consistent with other studies in the past two decades examining available data to determine rates of suicide for college students; these studies have consistently found that rates of suicide for college students are much lower than the general population—suggesting that being a college student is very likely a protective factor for suicide risk. An ongoing, longitudinal national surveillance system that identifies student death by suicide would contribute to the research agenda.

BOX 2-4
Rate of Student Death by Suicide from
the Big Ten Counseling Centers[a]

   Silverman et al (1997) conducted a comprehensive 10-year study at 13 Big Ten university campuses to get a more accurate understanding of deaths by suicide in college campuses. Silverman et al. (1997) collected data from 1980 to 1990, at which point the study stopped. In an effort to continue to understand suicide rates and trends in college campuses, the Big Ten Counseling Centers decided to continue to collect data on deaths by suicides in their campuses. Data collection resumed in 2003, and it continues to be collected, with some data entered retrospectively and some data entered prospectively.

   The current report uses an academic year time frame, which is defined as the 12-month period between September 1 to August 31. This reporting period is consistent to that used by Silverman et al. (1997), which more closely aligns to academic calendars in university campuses, which is relevant because the population studied is college students.

   The overall average suicide rate per 100,000 students is 5.60 for the years 2009 to 2018 in the Big Ten college campuses. This is lower than the rate calculated by Silverman et al. (1997), which was 7.5/100,000. Specifically, there was a

25.3 percent decrease in the suicide rate in Big Ten universities in 30 years from 1980-1990 to 2009-2018.

The rate of 5.60 is also lower than the U.S. population national average suicide rate of 14.2/100,000 based on 2018 data from the National Center for Health Statistics (NCHS) at the Centers for Disease Control and Prevention (CDC; Hedegaard, Curtin, and Warner, 2020). The 5.60/100,000 rate in college campuses is also lower than the average U.S. population suicide rate for age groups 15-24, 25-34, 35-44, and 45-54 for males and females, which was about 17/100,000 based on National Institute of Mental Health (NIMH) data from 2017 NIMH. In other words, the overall average suicide rate at Big Ten college campuses was 39.4 percent of the U.S. population national average. Additionally, the overall average suicide rate at Big Ten college campuses is 38.0 percent of the weighted average U.S. population suicide rate for college-aged individuals. Taken from a different perspective, the U.S. population national average suicide rate is about 254 percent higher than the average suicide rate in Big Ten universities.

---

[a] Thirteen Big Ten Universities participated in and contributed data for the study. The 13 participating universities were located in the MIdwest and Northeast in the United States in the following states: Illinois (Northwestern University, University of Illinois at Urbana–Champaign), Indiana (Indiana University, Purdue University), Iowa (University of Iowa), Michigan (Michigan State University, University of Michigan), Minnesota (University of Minnesota), Nebraska (University of Nebraska–Lincoln), New Jersey (Rutgers), Ohio (The Ohio State University), Pennsylvania (Pennsylvania State), and Wisconsin (University of Wisconsin–Madison).

CURRENT TRENDS IN SUBSTANCE USE IN HIGHER EDUCATION

Substance use remains a concern on colleges across the country given the effects illicit drugs and alcohol can have on the developing brains of young adults, many of which can have significant behavioral and cognitive consequences. The Substance Abuse and Mental Health Services Administration (SAMHSA) describes substance use disorders as occurring when they reach the level when "the recurrent use of alcohol and/or drugs causes clinically significant impairment, including health problems, disability, and failure to meet major responsibilities at work, school, or home" (SAMHSA, 2020c). Trends in use of substances, from recreational to abuse, are detailed in the sections below. Similar to mental health data, unless noted the data on substance use are self-reported.

Trends in Alcohol Use

In 2018, 60 percent of current U.S. college students reported past-month alcohol use, 28 percent reported binge drinking[8] in the past two weeks, and 10

---

[8] Binge drinking is defined as a pattern of drinking that brings blood alcohol concentration (BAC) levels to 0.08 percent. This typically occurs after four drinks for women and five drinks for men—in about two hours. High-intensity drinking is defined as alcohol intake at levels twice or more the threshold for binge drinking (NIAAA, 2018).

percent reported high-intensity drinking in the past two weeks. In the same year, 11 percent of full-time college students met clinical criteria for an alcohol use disorder (AUD) in the past year (SAMHSA, 2019d).

While alcohol use by college students remains high, data from several sources show that binge drinking among students has gone down over the past several years (see Table 2-6). For example, data from HMS show that self-reports of binge drinking "any time in the past two weeks" and "three or more times in the past 2 weeks" was down 18.16 percent and 28.09 percent, respectively, between 2013 and 2018. Similarly, self-reported data from ACHA-NCHA and clinical data from CCMH show a reduction in binge drinking among students between 2013 and 2018 (see Table 2-4).

One factor that may explain the drop in the percentage of students reporting binge drinking over time is a reduction in binge drinking among men. In a survey of the nation's college students and adults from ages 19 through 60, the authors found that prevalence of past-month alcohol consumption has declined modestly since 1980, when men had slightly higher use; the gender gap disappeared by 2000. Among college students, binge drinking has traditionally shown a significant gender difference, but a gradual long-term decline in binge drinking among college men since 1985 and little change among college women has narrowed the gap (in 2018, 32 percent of male college students binge drank compared to 27 percent of females) (Schulenberg et al., 2019).

However, another consistent finding has been that female students are more at risk for alcohol-related problems and have higher risk for meeting criteria for AUD (Clarke et al., 2013; Slutske, 2005). In 2018, 12 percent of male college students and 11 percent of female college students met criteria for AUD (SAMHSA, 2019d). An increase in the proportion of students with an AUD from 2017 to 2018 was significant among female students, but not male students.

TABLE 2-4 Comparison of Measures of Binge Drinking in Higher Education Students from Multiple Sources in 2013 and 2018

	Year		
Measures of Binge Drinking	Fall 2013 (%)	Fall 2018 (%)	% Change 2013-2018
CCMH: Binge drinking (Any in the past 2 weeks)[a]	41.1	37.4	- 8.10
CCMH: Binge drinking (3+ times in the past 2 weeks)[a]	12.6	10.1	- 19.84
HMS: Binge Drinking (Any in the past 2 weeks)[b]	45.7	37.4	- 18.16
HMS: Binge Drinking (3+ times in the past 2 weeks)[b]	17.8	12.8	- 28.09
NCHA: Binge Drinking (Any in the past 2 weeks)[c]	29.8	28.4	- 4.7
NCHA: Binge Drinking (3+ times in the past 2 weeks)[c]	9.2	7.0	- 23.9

[a]CCMH (clinical data); [b]HMS (general population data); [c]NCHA (general population data)
Sources: ACHA, 2014, 2018; CCMH, 2015, 2020a; HMN, 2007-2019.

College students are at increased risk for problematic patterns of alcohol use compared to their non-college-attending peers (Schulenberg et al., 2019). This has long been true. For example, although the 2001-2002 National Epidemiologic Survey on Alcohol and Related Conditions (NESARC) found that college students and their non-college peers consume alcohol at similarly heavy rates (Chen et al., 2004), college students had a higher prevalence of drinking and risk drinking than did their non-college peers. Nevertheless, the "rates of alcohol abuse and dependence are roughly equivalent for college and non-college individuals, and the development of alcohol-use disorders among young adults is more related to their living situation (e.g., at home with parents, on campus, off campus) than to college status itself" (Carter, Brandon, and Goldman, 2010; Dawson et al., 2004).

Furthermore, certain student groups are at higher risk for excessive alcohol use compared to their peers. For example, undergraduates have higher rates of binge drinking than graduate students (Cranford, Eisenberg, and Serras, 2009). A stable trend in college alcohol use since the 1980s is that white college students are the heaviest drinkers followed by Hispanic and Black students (Borsari, Murphy, and Barnett, 2007; Ham and Hope, 2003). Students who began drinking at an earlier age and come to college as established drinkers maintain or increase their drinking levels in their first year of college to levels well above their peers who were light drinkers or abstainers in high school (Borsari et al., 2007; Ham and Hope, 2003). College athletes drink alcohol more often, consume higher quantities of alcohol, and experience more negative alcohol-related consequences than non-athlete college students (Martens, Dams-O'Connor, and Beck, 2006). Similarly, involvement in a Greek organization (a fraternity or sorority) is consistently shown to be associated with heavier alcohol use compared to other students (Borsari et al., 2007; Ham and Hope, 2003).

College-level factors can also increase risk for excessive alcohol use among students. Students at 4-year colleges are more likely to binge drink compared to students at 2-year institutions. However, an important factor to consider is a student's living situation, since living with family has been shown to be a protective factor against excessive alcohol use. A larger proportion of students at 2-year colleges live with family compared to students at 4-year colleges (Velazquez et al., 2011). Regarding "dry" campuses, one study found that students had lower rates of alcohol use and binge drinking at schools that prohibited the use of alcohol on campus compared to schools that allowed alcohol use (Wechsler et al., 2001). Students were 30 percent less likely to be heavy episodic drinkers and 80 percent more likely to be abstainers at schools that prohibited alcohol use. The research literature shows a consistent association between a campus' proximity to alcohol outlets and increased alcohol use and related harms among college students and may be a more relevant risk factor than the geographic characteristics of the college itself (e.g., rural, urban) (Scribner et al., 2008; Weitzman et al., 2003).

Trends in Marijuana Use

Marijuana use by college students has increased over the past several years. Data from the HMS, CCMH, and ACHA-NCHA each show a roughly 30 percent increase in marijuana use by students between 2013 and 2018 (see Table 2-5). The primary driving force behind these increases is higher marijuana use by women in recent years.

Gender differences observed in past-year marijuana use prior to 2010 have vanished in 2018 (43 percent for college men and 42 percent for college women) as a result of steady levels of use among males and increasing use among females. Past-month vaping of marijuana is also following this trend, with use among male students increasing more modestly in recent years compared to females; in 2018, 13.1 percent of male college students vaped marijuana compared to 9.3 percent of females (Schulenberg et al., 2019). Daily marijuana use remains twice as high among college men (8.4 percent) compared to college women (4.3 percent).

Marijuana use among college students today may reflect new use patterns and products. The average level of tetrahydrocannabinol (THC), the main compound in marijuana responsible for mind-altering effects, in marijuana rose from 4 percent in 1995 to 15 percent in 2017 (NASEM, 2017). The rise in potency can be attributed to the different types of marijuana products on the market and new methods of production in recent years compared to decades ago. For example, extremely potent forms of marijuana concentrates are becoming more prevalent in the United States. These trends suggest that people who use marijuana may be more at risk of harms compared to previous years (Marconi et al., 2016; Murray et al., 2016; Volkow et al., 2016).

Trends in Prescription Medication Misuse

In 2018, 4 percent of full-time college students misused a prescription medication in the past month, a decrease from 5 percent in 2017, with stimulants being

TABLE 2-5 Comparison of Measures of Marijuana Use in Higher Education Students from Multiple Sources in 2013 and 2018

| Measures of Marijuana Use | Year | | |
	Fall 2013 (%)	Fall 2018 (%)	% Change 2013-2018
CCMH: Marijuana use (any in the past 2 weeks)[a]	20.1	25.8	28.36
CCMH: Marijuana use (3+ times in the past 2 weeks)[a]	11.4	15.3	34.21
HMS: Marijuana use (any time in the past month)[b]	16.1	21.5	33.5
ACHA-NCHA: Marijuana use (any use in the past 30 days)[c]	14.1	19.0	34.8

[a]CCMH (clinical data); [b]HMS (general population data); [c]NCHA (general population data)
Sources: ACHA, 2014, 2018; CCMH, 2015, 2020a; HMN, 2007-2019.

the most common prescription medication used non-medically among college students (McCabe et al., 2005a; SAMHSA, 2019d).[9] Risk factors for non-medical use of prescription stimulants include being male, white, a member of a Greek organization, and having a lower grade point average (Cranford et al., 2009). At the campus level, rates of non-medical stimulant use are higher at colleges in the Northeast region of the United States and at colleges with more competitive admission standards (McCabe et al., 2005a). Prescription drug misuse rarely occurs alone. Students who report non-medical stimulant use are also more likely to report alcohol, cigarette, marijuana, ecstasy, and cocaine use. Specifically, 70 percent of students who misused prescription stimulants in a national study were excessive drinkers and 68 percent used marijuana during the past month.

Opioid use (particularly heroin and synthetic opioid use) is less common in college students compared to their non-college-attending peers. In 2018, 1 percent of full-time college students in the United States used a prescription opioid non-medically in the past year (SAMHSA, 2019d). The college population has not been the focus of opioid research in recent years (McCabe et al., 2005b).

Impact of Substance Use on College Students

In 2004, the last year for which estimates are available, 599,000 college students were injured because of their alcohol use, 696,000 were hit or assaulted by another drinking college student, and 97,000 experienced a sexual assault or date rape perpetrated by another college student who had been drinking (Hingson, Zha, and Weitzman, 2009). Male students tend to experience more alcohol-related consequences that involve public deviance while consequences experienced by female students tend to be more personal; females also experience more dependence symptoms (Clarke et al., 2013; Ham and Hope, 2003).

A quarter of women in the United States have experienced sexual assault, and approximately half of those cases involve alcohol consumption by the perpetrator, victim, or both. Among college students, 22 percent report experiencing at least one incident of sexual assault (Mellins et al., 2017). In one study with a large

---

[9] From SAMHSA: Questions about past-year use and misuse in the 2018 NSDUH covered the following subcategories of stimulants: amphetamine products (Adderall®, Adderall® XR, Dexedrine®, Vyvanse®, generic dextroamphetamine, generic amphetamine/dextroamphetamine combinations, or generic extended-release A-71 amphetamine-dextroamphetamine combinations); methylphenidate products (Ritalin®, Ritalin® LA, Concerta®, Daytrana®, Metadate® CD, Metadate® ER, Focalin®, Focalin® XR, generic methylphenidate, generic extended-release methylphenidate, generic dexmethylphenidate, or generic extended-release dexmethylphenidate); anorectic (weight-loss) stimulants (Didrex®, benzphetamine, Tenuate®, diethylpropion, phendimetrazine, or phentermine); Provigil®; or any other prescription stimulant. Other prescription stimulants could include products similar to the specific stimulants listed previously. Since 2015, methamphetamine has not been included as a prescription stimulant. Questions were not asked about past-month stimulant use or misuse for the subtype categories.

college student sample, female students and gender nonconforming students reported the highest rates of sexual assault (28 percent for both), while 12.5 percent of men experienced assault. The most frequent correlate of experiencing assault was incapacitation as a result of alcohol and drug use (greater than 50 percent). Factors that increased risk for sexual assault included non-heterosexual identity, membership in a Greek organization, and binge drinking, among others. Drug- or alcohol-facilitated/incapacitated rape survivors are less likely to acknowledge their rape and therefore less likely to seek services or treatment (Walsh et al., 2016).

The 2019 Association of American Universities (AAU) Campus Climate Survey on Sexual Assault and Misconduct included 181,752 students from 33 colleges and universities, including 32 AAU member schools. The authors found that the "overall rate of non-consensual sexual contact by physical force or inability to consent since a respondent enrolled as a student at their school was 13 percent, with the rates for women and transgender, genderqueer, and non-binary (TGQN, defined as transgender, genderqueer, questioning or not listed) students being significantly higher than for men" (AAU, 2019).

American Psychiatric Association research shows consistently that the increasing intensity of marijuana use is associated with increasing risk for psychosis later in life (Marconi et al., 2016; Murray et al., 2016). Higher potency marijuana products and synthetic marijuana carry the most risk for psychotic outcomes. Marijuana use is also consistently shown to have a detrimental effect on cognitive function, and these consequences are magnified if use starts early in adolescence (Shrivastava, Johnson, and Tsuang, 2011). Further, a robust meta-analysis concluded that marijuana use is a significant predictor of developing depression, suicidal ideation, and experiencing a suicide attempt (Gobbi et al., 2019). Overall, the risk for these mental health outcomes remains moderate to low among young adults using marijuana. However, the increasing numbers of young people using marijuana creates a larger population who could develop depression or suicidality attributable to marijuana use and exacerbate the mental health situation among college students in the United States. Regarding the acute impacts of marijuana use, research is consistent in showing that marijuana use causes acute impairment of learning and memory, attention, and working memory, but whether there is enduring neuropsychological impairment is less clear (Volkow et al., 2016).

COMORBIDITY BETWEEN MENTAL HEALTH AND SUBSTANCE USE IN HIGHER EDUCATION

"Comorbidity" is the term used to describe the presence of two or more illnesses at the same time. According to the National Institute on Drug Abuse (NIDA), comorbidities "can occur at the same time or one after the other. Comorbidity also implies interactions between the illnesses that can worsen the course of both" (NIDA, 2020c). It is also possible that the presence of one condition may contribute to the development of another. Individuals with mental illness, for example, may use substances as a coping mechanism to deal with the symptoms of this disorder, even though substance use can also exacerbate underlying conditions. Similarly, the repeated use of drugs or alcohol can affect the way the brain works, which can increase an individual's susceptibility to developing mental health issues (NIDA, 2020c).

The use of substances in adolescents and young adults poses a particular set of risks, as these years are critical to brain development. In fact, research shows that "early drug use is a strong risk factor for later development of substance use disorders, and it may also be a risk factor for the later occurrence of other mental illnesses" (NIDA, 2020a). While this is not a causal link, adolescence and young adulthood are times when both mental illness and substance use disorders are likely to begin.

While not specific to college students, for young adults, approximately 8.9 million individuals aged 18-25 had any mental illness (AMI) in the past year, and 5.1 million had a past-year substance use disorder (SUD). In this age group, 2.4 million had both AMI and an SUD in the past year (approximately 7.2 percent of young adults). In that group, 43.8 percent received substance use or mental health care in 2018. Of that group, 37.9 percent received only mental health care, 3.7 percent received care for both, and 2.0 percent for substance abuse only (CBHSQ, 2019).

Approximately 1.7 million young adults aged 18-25 had a severe mental illness coinciding with an SUD, or 1.7 of adults in this age group. In this age group, 60.1 percent received either mental health care or substance use treatment. Within this group that received treatment, 52.8 received only mental health care, 5.8 percent received treatment for both, and 1.5 percent received substance use treatment only (CBHSQ, 2019). The rates of parallel treatment for comorbid conditions, however, do not align with the latest research findings suggesting that treating mental health and substance use disorders in concert can provide longer-lasting effects.

There are other types of comorbidity in addition to mental illness and substance use. Different mental health disorders can occur together—comorbid anxiety and depression, for example—and they can co-occur with physical health disorders—depression and diabetes, for instance (OPA, 2020). The links between mental health, substance use, and physical health may tie into an individual's environment from infancy through young adulthood. A multitude of factors can contribute to the development of comorbid issues: "The interaction between childhood activities and biology could affect brain development and—ultimately—social, behavioral, academic, health, and other outcomes" (OPA, 2020).

3

Environments to Support
Wellbeing for All Students

Definitions of wellbeing vary, but for the purposes of this report, as described in previous chapters, wellbeing is a holistic concept referring to both physical and mental health. Balanced nutrition, exercise, sleep, and proper hygiene, coupled with access to medical care for temporary and chronic conditions, supports physical wellbeing.

Support for student wellbeing does not mean that students will not experience stress or difficult periods. It does not mean that colleges and universities are responsible for ensuring that students avoid all emotional discomfort and that on-campus treatment is available for all needs. What higher education can do, with its focus on academic development and through its actions and policies, is inform lifelong behaviors, both healthy and risky, that can develop during this time. While colleges and universities do not need to have health services that address all possible student needs, they do have an obligation to make students aware of the resources available to them, including academic support, health-related services, and wellbeing programs. In the event there are clinical health services available, students should have access to transparent information about the scope of services, cost and fees, and other community resources when a licensed provider is needed (See Chapter 4 for additional information on clinical services).

Institutions of higher education have increased their attention to student wellbeing over recent decades. This shift aligns with a movement in broader U.S. society beginning in the early 1990s, when the federal government began to increase efforts related to health and wellbeing in the workplace with *Healthy People 2000*.[1] While higher education's role in supporting student wellbeing has incrementally

---

[1] See: https://spark.adobe.com/page/BmX0QbGmKRJ1d.

increased over the better part of the past century, documentation from the past decade includes the integration of wellbeing into higher education: *Considering Wellbeing, and its Connection to Learning and Civic Engagement, as Central to the Mission of Higher Education* (2013); the Okanagan Charter (*Okanagan Charter: An international charter for health promoting universities and colleges*, 2015); and The Council for the Advancement of Standards within Higher Education's cross-functional framework for advancing health and wellbeing (Travia et al., 2019). These documents can serve as an overarching framework for wellbeing in higher education to span "health, wellbeing, flourishing, and thriving of college students in the context of a healthy community" (Travia et al., 2019).

This chapter covers broad, campus-wide efforts to support overall student wellbeing and success. It also profiles specific populations of students and provides insights into how higher education can support students across all of their identities. These descriptions also include information on populations of students more likely to have been exposed to trauma and harm perpetuated against them. Finally, as students often identify with multiple groups, the profiles make note of the ways that individuals with intersecting identities might benefit from additional support. Recognizing students' full identities contributes to educational and training environments that support that wellbeing of all students.

SUPPORTING THE GENERAL STUDENT POPULATION THROUGH WELLBEING AND WELLBEING STRATEGIES

Many campuses offer wellbeing resources and programs open to all students. These wellbeing efforts, which are not intended to replace clinical services or grow needed clinical service capacity, do provide education and skill-building aimed at preventing and mitigating less severe instances of stress that can lead to more serious mental health issues. For some students who have not had access to education related to general health, exposure to information on nutrition, physical activity, sleep, and other factors that contribute to wellbeing may be the first step to developing and maintaining healthy habits.

Wellbeing programs on campus employ a variety of approaches, and the availability of services varies considerably depending on existing funding, staff, and type of institution. For example, the National Institute on Alcoholism and Alcohol Abuse (NIAAA)[2] offers a range of evidence-based strategies and interventions—sorted by level of efficacy and cost—that institutions of higher education can use to develop and deploy wellbeing activities that support efforts to reduce alcohol use among college students. The suggested approaches include skills training, brief motivational interventions, and personalized feedback interventions (NIAAA, 2019). At the campus level, colleges and universities can raise awareness about available services, launch campaigns to reduce stigma related to

---

[2] See: https://www.niaaa.nih.gov.

mental health and associated services, and ensure that policies, including those prohibiting bullying, harassment, and assault, promote mental health and wellbeing. Colleges and universities might also create opportunities for students to build community and peer support and develop healthy connections with faculty and staff. At the individual student level, workshops, seminars, and other events may provide them the opportunity to alleviate stress, develop mechanisms for processing challenges, and learn about other ways to adopt a healthy lifestyle, including exercise, meditation, nutrition, sleep, and other health-related behaviors.

Campus Programs and Activities

Pre-orientation materials, orientation events, and workshops held at the institutional, department, or program level are channels through which colleges and universities can transmit information about wellbeing services. However, for students enrolled at community colleges, graduate programs, and professional schools, the introduction to campus may not include the same volume of events as residential, undergraduate programs. Graduate and professional students may only receive information on their school or department without guidance to the campus as a whole.

As part of orientation, some campuses provide students with mental and emotional health screenings as a way to understand important signals related to overall health and gain a baseline understanding of their existing wellbeing. While these screenings are not diagnostic, may be prone to over-estimating prevalence rates (see Chapter 2), and cannot replace the evaluation of a licensed professional, early screenings can provide students with an understanding of what warning signs for distress look like in themselves as well as others. Screening sessions can also provide students with information about health and wellbeing services on campus and connect them to national resources (SAMHSA, 2018).

Beyond helping students build individual skills, colleges and universities may also support student wellbeing through community and group activities. Student-led groups can take many forms and focus on a range of interests, including academic, athletic, social, religious, and spiritual affiliation, community service, and professional interests, as well as groups based around student traits or identities. Building connections with peers can alleviate loneliness and provide students with a sense of belonging on campus. These groups can also help students with opportunities to reduce stress and to learn new skills, and they can serve as venues to continue activities and hobbies they may have enjoyed prior to enrolling in their program. While student-led groups may provide valuable assistance, and in some cases informal support, the administration may not be aware such services are being offered.

Campus Mental Health Services

In addition to orientation programs and student groups, colleges and universities often employ other strategies to support students and inform them about mental health services. Campaigns that reduce stigma around mental health issues and challenges can normalize help-seeking behavior and encourage students to access services that may suit their needs (e.g., a stress management workshop or in-person counseling). (See Box 3-1 that describes some current national efforts to address stigma against mental health and highlights some examples of efforts under way at individual institutions). Colleges may work with visible and well-known offices on campuses (e.g., student services, financial aid, residential life, and recreational facilities) to host workshops and provide resources on nonacademic skills that can support student mental health. In the event that a campus experiences a student death by suicide, there may be additional support

---

BOX 3-1
Efforts to Address Stigma Against Mental Illness

The stigma associated with mental health conditions can serve as a significant barrier to students with mental health disabilities getting the help they are entitled to under the law. A nationwide survey conducted by Salzer and colleagues of 190 current and 318 former college students with mental health disabilities found that concern about stigma undermined students' willingness to seek accommodations. The researchers found that 30 percent of the students surveyed did not want to disclose their mental health disability out of concern that they would be stigmatized by teachers, while 20 percent "were fearful of being stigmatized by other students" (Salzer et al., 2008).

There are several national initiatives aimed at reducing the stigma associated with mental illness. For example, mtvU and the Jed Foundation's Half of Us[a] campaign aims "to initiate a public dialogue to raise awareness about the prevalence of mental health issues and connect students to the appropriate resources to get help." The campaign website features the stories of celebrities from music, television, and movies who share their personal experiences with mental illness and substance use in an effort to normalize open dialogue about these issues and to encourage help-seeking behavior among students. Similarly, the Bring Change 2 Mind effort, co-founded by actress Glenn Close, strives "to end the stigma and discrimination surrounding mental illness." To do so, they create "multimedia campaigns, curate storytelling movements, and develop youth programs to encourage a diverse cultural conversation around mental health." The Bring Change 2 Mind 2018 impact evaluation found that the effort has had broad reach, with its public service announcements reaching roughly 6 billion people across a range of media. Additional evaluation of these efforts would shed important light on their impact and reach on college and university campuses.

sought, prevention and awareness services provided, and questions around communication.

Most importantly, institutions offer mental health supports through counseling centers, which have been found to be effective in supporting emotional wellness for students. McAleavey et al. (2017) conducted randomized controlled trials (RCTs) to evaluate the effectiveness of psychotherapy in a large (N =9895) sample of clients in university counseling centers. The authors found that while there are areas for improvement, in general, "across several different problem areas, routine psychotherapy provided substantial benefit, particularly to clients in the most distress." In its 2017 annual report, CCMH reported that students who came to counseling centers in 2012-2017 with "high levels of initial distress" reported that their distress level decreased from 2.65 to 1.8 on the CCAPS Distress Index after 10 sessions (CCMH, 2018).

Individual campuses have also launched efforts to reduce stigma against mental health. For example, as described in the report, the California Community Colleges have used a suite of six online, interactive training simulations from Kognito, a for-profit entity, to reduce stigma and engage faculty, staff, and students in supporting those exhibiting signs of distress. The result was a 73 percent increase in the number of students that faculty, staff, and students referred to mental health services across 113 campuses (Kognito, 2016; Sontag-Padilla et al., 2018c).

Some efforts to reduce stigma against mental health are explicitly considering how heightened stigma in communities of color can undermine the mental health and wellbeing of BIPOC students. For example, as described in the report, Therapy for Black Girls is a free online service that aims both to reduce the stigma of treatment and help African American women, including students, find a local community-based therapist. Efforts that take such an intersectional approach are critical to supporting the improved mental health and wellbeing of BIPOC students, however, additional research is needed to better understand how campuses can most effectively support students of color.

Increasing the number of mental health professionals who are BIPOC can also help reduce the stigma associated with mental health treatment among BIPOC students. SAMHSA's Historically Black Colleges and Universities Center for Excellence (HBCU-CFE) in Behavioral Health is specifically designed to increase the number of students at HBCUs who pursue careers in behavioral health. The program's activities "emphasize education, awareness, and preparation for careers in mental and substance use disorder treatment, including addressing opioid use disorder treatment, serious mental illness (SMI) (including First Episode Psychosis (FEP)), and suicide prevention" (SAMHSA, 2020b).

---

[a] See: http://www.halfofus.com/about-half-of-us.

Supporting Students Online

Today's students have had greater exposure to online and virtual environments than previous generations. These "digital natives" not only have greater exposure to tools and programs, but also have experienced more of their life through social media and virtual outlets. As the pressure on mental health services on campus has increased, colleges have sought other technology-enabled methods for supporting students. These include mental health applications and virtual health and wellbeing tools (Kern et al., 2018), not to be confused with telehealth, which are one-on-one services offered directly by a mental health provider through virtual means. These mental health applications have become particularly popular during the COVID pandemic. For example, numerous online programs to support mental health have become popular in the higher education setting, including several that provide digital behavioral health care, specifically online programs to support treatment for depression, anxiety, stress, and resilience for college students.

While colleges and universities may seek virtual health and wellbeing tools (separate from telehealth and distance therapy services), the evidence base regarding their effectiveness remains limited. Estimates suggest that of the 325,000 available emerging digital health technologies, as many as 12,000 focus on mental health (ADAA, 2020).

Although many community colleges were more likely to provide a form of online education prior to COVID-19, there has been little done to understand how they use virtual tools to educate and support students. Additional research on support mechanisms, from general wellbeing to more specific mental health, for primarily virtual students would provide a great service to the community college community, as well as others turning to hybrid and virtual models during the pandemic (Chiauzzi et al., 2011).

There have been several studies of the efficacy of online interventions for reducing stress, depression, and anxiety in students. Farrer et al. (2013) conducted a systematic review of technological interventions targeting certain mental health and related problems in university settings. The authors noted that "technological interventions targeting certain mental health and related problems offer promise for students in university settings. The data suggest that technology-based CBT may be particularly useful in targeting anxiety and, to a lesser extent, depressive symptoms in interventions targeting both depression and anxiety." Similarly, Davies, Morriss, and Glazebrook (2014) found that computer-delivered and web-based interventions designed to improve depression, anxiety, and psychological well-being of university students can be "effective in improving students' depression, anxiety, and stress outcomes when compared to inactive controls." However, the authors cautioned that these interventions need to be "trialed on more heterogeneous student samples and would benefit from user evaluation."

In another related study of these interventions and applications, Conley et al. (2019) noted that additional research may be needed to assess the effectiveness, including cost-effectiveness, of the types of interventions and their components; how they are delivered, including through which types of technological devices; and the target populations. Lattie, Lipson, and Eisenberg (2019) noted the need for further research to ascertain the effective elements of digital mental health tools, and Harrer et al. (2019) added that research is also needed to examine the "student subsets for which Internet-based interventions are most effective and to explore ways to increase treatment effectiveness." Virtual platforms can also provide opportunities outside of the digital classroom for students who attend higher education in hybrid or online models to meet and interact with other students. In fact, virtual environments can provide a place of connection for all students to share stories and form a support network. For example, PhD Balance[3] is an online community developed by graduate students to share narratives about mental and emotional health struggles and share resources. Other virtual spaces, notably for students who have not developed connections on campus, can provide other channels to develop relationships and find support based on their interests. #BlackandSTEM, for example, is an online community that uses Twitter to connect a community of Black professionals, students, and teachers across the country (Ireland et al., 2018; Montgomery, 2018).

The online environment has been shown to impact students' emotional health. Research indicates, for example, that adolescents receiving positive reactions to their social media presence have higher self-esteem and are more satisfied with life (Ahn, 2011). On the other hand, social media that is perceived to be negative, including social rejection and cyberbullying, can negatively affect an individual's emotional state (Chou and Edge, 2011; NASEM, 2020). Social media may also bias and skew perceptions of normative behavior ranging from body image, substance use, socializing and partying, and other behaviors than can enhance feelings of loneliness, decrease a feeling of belonging or welcome, and limit connection to others (Huang et al., 2014; Zhu, 2017).

Another concern is that students may feel unsure about how to connect with other students who share posts that include distressing information or suggest that the account holder may be experiencing difficulties. The Jed Foundation and the Clinton Foundation created a guide for students with information about identifying warning signs, guidance on how to respond, and national resources for reference (Jed Foundation and Clinton Foundation, 2014).

Online dating apps also have the potential to threaten both psychological and physical health. Individuals who use these apps can avoid vulnerable situations by developing safety protocols that include meeting with individuals in public settings, letting a friend or trusted individual know about the event, and limiting the amount of personal information and/or images shared in advance (Breitschuh and Göretz, 2019; Wong et al., 2020).

Finally, many students do not have a full understanding of the terms of service, data sharing policies, and privacy guidelines to which they agree when they use

---

[3] Additional information is available at https://www.phdbalance.com (accessed August 17, 2020).

apps and social media. Providing guidance about the impact of social media on emotional health, an understanding of how algorithms operate to promote content, and privacy concerns regarding user data can help students foster safe and productive relationships with the online environment (Brandtzaeg, Pultier, and Moen, 2018; Obar and Oeldorf-Hirsch, 2020; Sarikakis and Winter, 2017).

PROVIDING SUPPORT FOR SPECIFIC STUDENT POPULATIONS

Many institutions of higher education have offices, groups, and/or staff on campus dedicated to working with specific groups of students. While these populations are described in isolation, students can and often do hold multiple overlapping identities, such as a first-generation student who is Black, Indigenous or a Person of Color (BIPOC) and a veteran. While this chapter primarily focuses on population-level programs and wellbeing services, the sections on specific populations below do include some information on ways these groups may exhibit certain characteristics related to mental health and wellbeing, reported rates of mental health issues, differences in access or rates of mental health utilization, and other clinical services covered in greater detail in Chapter 4.

Black, Indigenous, and Students of Color

As noted in Chapter 2, the proportion of students who are Black, African American, Hispanic, Asian, Pacific Islanders, Native American/Alaska Native, and multiple-race non-Hispanic is projected to increase in the coming years. BIPOC students often have intersecting identities, including first-generation status, having a disability, having insecure documentation status, or being a survivor of trauma. BIPOC students are also more likely to be part-time students, work while a student, live with dependents, and come from families with lower annual incomes (Espinosa et al., 2019).

BIPOC students, compared to the student body as a whole, are more likely to have experienced conditions that impact their health, education, and development, such as experiences resulting from systemic racism and oppression (Ingram and Wallace, 2018), limited access to health care and health insurance (including mental health); food insecurity; domestic violence; housing insecurity and eviction; bankruptcy; interruption of education due to relocation; and exposure to environmental health hazards (Jury et al., 2017; Metcalfe and Neubrander, 2016; Sohn, 2017). These additional factors, when present, should not be misinterpreted as implying that BIPOC students do not have potential and responsibilities in terms of academic achievement, leadership capabilities, or contributions to campus. Rather, institutions of higher education, and especially those that are predominantly white institutions, need to recognize that the pervasive effects of systemic racism and sexism, including inequality in K-12 education, can coalesce with college policies and practices in ways that compromise postsecondary academic resilience (Jack, 2019). As students from these groups continue to enter higher education at higher rates, colleges and universities hoping to support students from admission to graduation may consider investing in programs and services that provide support specific to these students.

One such program, The Husky Promise, was designed to support low-income students in Washington state, as defined by the requirements for Pell Grants or the Washington State Need Grant (Cauce, 2019). Through this program, students could attend any of three University of Washington campuses without paying tuition. Students also received financial aid to help with the cost of attendance as well, such as rent, food, etc. Cauce (2019) notes that original projections were that about 5,000 students a year would attend the University of Washington through the Husky Promise. "Ten years later, almost 40,000 students have availed themselves of the program, which covers students for up to 5 years, and today we have about 10,000 Husky Promise students across our three campuses."

Similarly, University of North Carolina (UNC), through its Carolina Covenant program, offers students whose family has an adjusted gross income (AGI) that is at or below 200 percent of the poverty guideline financial aid to attend and graduate from UNC-Chapel Hill (UNC, 2020). The program is designed to "communicate a clear, simple message of predictability of financial aid for low-income students, and promises that low-income students can graduate debt-free." The Covenant program, which has been found to contribute to the academic success of these students, incorporates a campus-wide support network and commitment to student success. A mentoring program is also a central component of the support network (Ort, 2020).

Understanding and recognizing the biases that students from these groups may face is only the first step in establishing programs aimed at fostering wellbeing in these student communities. Faculty and staff recognition of how students who are BIPOC respond to stress and react in ways distinct from the majority-white student body can reduce microaggressions and actions that create hostile environments (Ryu and Thompson, 2018). Institutions of higher education can offer staff, faculty, and all others who interact with students training and focus on developing skills, knowledge, and attitudes to understand ways to identify racist behavior, correct biased policies, and provide all students with support (Ryu and Thompson, 2018).

In addition to providing culturally competent programs and services to students, colleges and universities may consider how they communicate, raise awareness, and reduce stigma around mental health specifically for students who are BIPOC. Research has shown that the presentation of symptoms can differ based on racial and ethnic backgrounds, as can engaging in help-seeking behaviors that differ from those of cisgender, heteronormative white men (Ryu and Thompson, 2018). This can make it difficult for those trained to recognize mental health symptoms based on cisgender, heteronormative white men in students who are BIPOC and make it less likely they will seek treatment (Ryu and Thompson, 2018).

Having health professionals on campus who recognize, support, and treat students from all backgrounds can help lower some of the barriers for students who are BIPOC. This may include staff at the general or primary health clinic who can recognize signs of mental health issues as well as processes that allow students to move between physical and mental health services. Research has demonstrated that biases in providers, notably along the lines of race and gender, can impact the efficacy of diagnoses and treatment plans for patients (Chapman et al., 2013; Green et al., 2007; IOM, 2003; Obermeyer et al., 2019). Actively and consistently addressing the systemic and institutional biases that exist in policies and in individuals can ameliorate the harm done to students from underrepresented groups and contribute to a more supportive environment.

This section, while it provides insight into the ways that students who are BIPOC could benefit from intentional support, does not provide an in-depth review of how these issues vary across different racial and ethnic groups. While on a statistical basis, students who are BIPOC may more often be first-generation students or less represented on campus, this is not always the case. Building programs and services that are equitable and inclusive means recognizing how higher education at times dictates a one-size-fits-all approach that colleges and universities can now work to undo and create campuses that support all students. Listening to individual students and how they characterize their experience will allow them to bring their full selves and thrive in their whole identity (Cook-Sather, 2018; Cropps and Esters, 2018; García and Henderson, 2014; Lehmann, Davies, and Lauren, 2000; Rasheem et al., 2018; Reddick and Pritchett, 2015; Syed et al., 2011).

Students with Disabilities and Disabled Students[4]

In 2015-2016, 19 percent of undergraduate (3,755,000) and 12 percent of postgraduate (423,000) students reported having a disability (Snyder et al.,

---

[4] The committee would like to acknowledge that the National Center for Disability and Journalism recognizes that different communities prefer the use of person-first (persons with disabilities) and identity-first (disabled persons) terminology. According to the NCDJ:

Background: The phrased "disabled people" is an example of identity-first language (in contrast to people-first language). It is the preferred terminology in Great Britain and by a growing number of U.S. disability activists. Syracuse University's Disability Cultural Center says, "The basic reason behind members of (some disability) groups' dislike for the application of people-first language to themselves is that they consider their disabilities to be inseparable parts of who they are." For example, they prefer to be referred to as "autistic," "blind," or "disabled." Several U.S. disabilities groups have always used identity-first terms, specifically the culturally deaf community and the autistic rights community.

NCDJ Recommendation: Ask the disabled person or disability organizational spokesperson about their preferred terminology. If that is not possible, use people-first language (NCDJ, 2018).

2019),[5] an increase over the past 20 years from 5.3 percent (892,000) of under-graduates and 3.2 percent (89,000) graduate or first-professional students (NCES, 1999, Table 211). Within this group, there is a higher percentage of undergraduate students who are also veterans (26 percent) than those who have not served in the military (19 percent) and higher percentage of students aged 30 and over (23 per-cent) than those aged 15-23 (18 percent) (Snyder et al., 2019a).

For students, the disability designation can be for a physical, behavioral, or learning disability.[6] The 1990 Americans with Disabilities Act (ADA) defines disability in the context of higher education as "a physical or mental impairment that substantially limits one or more major life activities, a person who has a history or record of such an impairment, or a person who is perceived by others as having such an impairment" (DOJ, 1990). ADA recognizes five categories of impairments that require mental health diagnoses: anxiety disorder, depres-sion, bipolar disorder, schizophrenia, and other psychological disorders. In the context of higher education, a mental health disability is defined as "a persistent psychological or psychiatric disorder, emotional or mental illness that adversely affects educational performance." To comply with ADA, campuses must pro-vide accommodations commensurate with the range of disabilities that students experience. Disabilities may be long-term and chronic, but ADA also covers short-term disability for surgery, trauma, or other medical conditions (including pregnancy). Given that students with disabilities are not a monolith, faculty and staff supporting these students will want to approach mental health and identity issues with sensitivity (Iarovici, 2014).

The percentage of students diagnosed with mental health disabilities is in-creasing. These students can face challenges in receiving necessary accommo-dations because their disability is often less visible and poorly understood by the campus community, including by faculty, than physical disabilities (e.g., blindness, deafness) (Condra et al., 2015). According to a report by the National

---

[5] From ED: Students with disabilities are those who reported that they had one or more of the fol-lowing conditions: blindness or visual impairment that cannot be corrected by wearing glasses; hear-ing impairment (e.g., deaf or hard of hearing); orthopedic or mobility impairment; speech or language impairment; learning, mental, emotional, or psychiatric condition (e.g., serious learning disability, depression, ADD, or ADHD); or other health impairment or problem.

From the American Community Survey 2017: The American Community Survey (ACS) estimates the overall rate of people with disabilities in the US population in 2016 was 12.8 percent. The percentage of those with a disability in the US civilian population slowly increased from 11.9 percent in 2010 to 12.8 percent in 2016. See: https://disabilitycompendium.org/sites/default/files/user-uploads/2017_An-nualReport_2017_FINAL.pdf.

[6] According to the Department of Education, students with disabilities are those who reported that they had one or more of the following conditions: blindness or visual impairment that cannot be cor-rected by wearing glasses; hearing impairment (e.g., deaf or hard of hearing); orthopedic or mobility impairment; speech or language impairment; learning, mental, emotional, or psychiatric condition (e.g., serious learning disability, depression, ADD, or ADHD); or other health impairment or problem See: https://ies.ed.gov/ncser/definition.asp.

Council on Disability (2017, p. 15), "College faculty, staff, and administrators need training to 1) identify and support students with mental health disabilities and 2) responsibly provide disability-related modifications and accommodations as required under federal disability laws." A survey of 76 practitioner and 148 students, carried out by the National Alliance on Mental Illness (NAMI), identified a range of practices that "colleges can engage in to enhance the inclusion, retention, and graduation of students with mental health disabilities" (NCD, 2017a)." Among those named as promising practices by respondents were:

- Making efforts to reduce stigma associated with mental health disabilities, which may take the form of staff workshops and professional development, faculty outreach, the efforts of student groups and student-led programs (such as those provided by Active Minds and NAMI), campus-wide events or activities, and work with external groups, such as NAMI (see Box 3-1)
- Locating offices for mental health services thoughtfully in order to provide students with confidential access when necessary or desired
- Creating a campus culture that normalizes discussion of mental health as a component of the wellness for the entire campus through the actions and statements of campus leaders
- Hiring case managers to provide resources to students in distress
- Educating faculty in how to identify students in need and refer them to campus support services and resources
- Entering into partnerships with community resources in the larger health care system when on campus resources are limited

Table 3-1 from the 2017 National Council on Disability report shows the percentage of students and practitioners who named certain practices as best practices in mental health services.

Disabled students may also benefit from additional support and programs that intersect with other identities as a means of preventing potential problems with loneliness and isolation (Iarovici, 2014). According to one report, "students with disabilities were also more likely to be from an ethnic minority group than students without disabilities, to identify as biracial or multiracial, and to identify as gay or bisexual" (Iarovici, 2014). This suggests that peer group and community activities that support students in their identities across the lines of race, ethnicity, gender, and sexual gender minorities may benefit from deliberate efforts to reach students with those identities who are also disabled.

Feelings of social isolation and lack of connection experienced by students with disabilities align with other mental health risks, such as developing a substance use disorder. Indeed, research has found that students with disabilities were more likely to engage in risky substance use (Iarovici, 2014), with the

TABLE 3-1 Percentage of Practitioners and Students Who Named Certain Practices as Best Practices in Mental Health Services

Practice	% of Practitioners	% of Students
Training/anti-stigma/outreach	26	65
Increased access	21	19
Student engagement	17	15
Faculty support/training	14	6
Crisis response/behavioral intervention teams	7	0
Pedagogy/universal design	5	0
Culturally competent practices	5	0
Technology access	5	0
Intracollege collaboration	2	0
Suicide prevention	2	0
More data availability	2	0
Skills training	2	0
Policy	2	0
Emotional support animals	2	0

Source: NCD, 2017a.

rate of substance misuse among students with a disability ranging from 14 to 65 percent across all disabilities (Casseus et al., 2020). Given the complexity and breadth of the types of disabilities experienced by students, there is a need to understand substance use disorders with greater nuance. Overall, the research on substance use in the population of students with disabilities remains limited, and additional research[7] would help provide insight into rates of prevalence and appropriate mechanisms to support students with disabilities to completion of their degree program.

First-Generation Students

As enrollment in higher education has continued to rise, there has been growing attention to students who are the first in their family to attend college or whose parent or guardian did not attain a bachelor's degree. For these students, the important factor regarding mental health is that they often lack the benefits of family members who can provide institutional knowledge on how to navigate the bureaucracy of higher education and its services. First-generation students can benefit from additional support related to the barriers related to finances, academics, and sense of belonging (PNPI, 2020a).

---

[7] Chapter 6 discusses open research questions that need to be answered.

Even though first-generation students come from all backgrounds, they are more likely to be BIPOC or have an identity that has been historically excluded from higher education. In 2012, 41 percent of Black and 61 percent of Latinx students identified as first-generation, in contrast to 25 percent of white and Asian-American students (PNPI, 2020a). First-generation students can differ from continuing-generation students, who have at least one parent with a postsecondary degree, in other distinct demographic and socioeconomic characteristics, too (see Table 3-2).

Developing specific communication strategies for first-generation students to raise awareness about the availability, cost, location, and purpose of programs and services available through campus wellbeing, general health, and mental health offerings can promote wellbeing and college completion (Wang and Joshi, 2018). Many first-generation students may benefit from programs and services embedded in places they are likely to visit in their daily interactions, such as academic buildings or community centers, or might visit for other health reasons, such as a general health clinic or women's health clinics. Extended hours later in the evening or on the weekends and available day care might also help first-generation students with dependents and those who work full time (Wang and Joshi, 2018).

Mentoring programs may also be useful in supporting the social, emotional, and academic needs of first-generation students (Plaskett et al., 2018). As an example, Cornell University's College of Agriculture and Life Sciences (CALS) peer mentoring program, for example, is designed for incoming first-generation students and was developed "to help students feel more closely connected to the campus environment and to help them bridge gaps in academic success and psychological well-being." The program, which pairs upperclassmen with incoming students based on majors and general demographic information, was found to be successful in improving academic performance and supporting psychological wellbeing. The 60 first-year students who fully engaged with the mentoring programs earned grade point averages that averaged 0.61 higher than those who did not. As evaluators of

TABLE 3-2 Comparison of Characteristics between First-Generation and Continuing-Generation Students in 2015-2016

Characteristic	First-Generation Students	Continuing-Generation Students
Age 30 or above	28 percent	16 percent
Has dependents	30 percent	16 percent
Female	60 percent	52 percent
Median annual parental income among dependent students	$41,000	$90,000

Source: PNPI, 2020a.

the program noted, "part of a student's academic success is making sure they are having a good psychological experience on campus....Providing academic guidance as well as social support helps students to navigate the often difficult, but important, journey of collegiate life" (Cornell University, 2020).

International Students and Students without Documentation

In 2017, 1,000,722 students were classified as non-resident aliens, accounting for 5.1 percent of total enrolled student population, 0.3 percent of the undergraduate population, and 14.2 percent at the postbaccalaureate level (NCES, 2017). While this group of students is often categorized with the blanket term "international students," the label does not provide the nuance to all the nationalities and backgrounds present at U.S. colleges and universities. While this grouping does not disaggregate between the many different cultures present, there are some common trends for institutions of higher education to acknowledge in the support of international students.

The relocation and life change that international students experience may contribute to culture shock upon arrival on campus (Iarovici, 2014). While many colleges and universities have offices and or staff dedicated to supporting international students, assistance beyond logistical and administrative support can ease the transition for those students navigating a new country. Support groups that provide a sense of community and a welcoming environment to those from their country of origin can provide international students with opportunities to develop social connections and a sense of belonging on campus and learn the nuances of life on a U.S. campus. These groups may include other international students who can share stories about their experience and normalize challenges or they may provide international students the opportunity to build connections to students with U.S. citizenship.

There are important considerations for colleges and universities to attend to while providing support for international students. The concepts of wellbeing and mental health, for example, may differ considerably depending on the students' country of origin, and international students utilize counseling services at lower rates and are less likely to return after an intake appointment (Alexander and Iarovici, 2018). Colleges may consider offering sessions on an as-needed basis or in groups settings that convene outside of the counseling center to create settings that feel more familiar and comfortable to students who feel less comfortable with the U.S. presentation of mental health and wellbeing services (Alexander and Iarovici, 2018). Providers and staff may also consider adapting counseling styles and programming to fit the expectations and the interests of international students (Iarovici, 2014).

In addition to international students, there is a population of undocumented students attending U.S. colleges and universities. Some 47 percent of undocumented students came to the United States before age 12, and 39 percent came between the ages of 13 to 21 (Feldblum et al., 2020). In 2018, the American Community Survey estimated there were approximate 450,000 students without documentation enrolled in higher education, accounting for about 2 percent of all students (Feldblum et al., 2020). Of students without documentation, a subset of 216,000 students (1 percent of all students) are eligible for Deferred Action for Childhood Arrivals (DACA) status. Conducting research and collecting data on undocumented individuals is difficult given that they may not wish to participate in any activity that could reveal their citizenship status and jeopardize themselves or their family. In terms of supporting students without documentation, there are a number of barriers to consider. Students may avoid academic, financial, health, and other campus services in fear of exposing themselves or family's undocumented status. Students without documentation may also have less familial financial stability, as their relatives may not have labor protections if they are also undocumented or live in another country. The students themselves also may not qualify or be willing to pursue the process to receive financial aid (including work study funding), scholarships, or employment. Students without documentation may also be first-generation students, who may be less likely to understand how tuition and fees may grant them access to free or low-cost health care options (Perez et al., 2009; Suárez-Orozco et al., 2015).

Beyond providing support that aligns with the needs of international students and students without documentation, there are also unique stressors that can affect their lives and mental health, as well as their ability to pursue their studies. Government regulations related to immigration, travel restrictions, and visas can create urgent situations for international and undocumented students. In the event of potential or pending policy changes, colleges and universities can rely on student services, immigration support staff, and centers for international students to provide updates and resources to students. These regulations may also impact their ability to pursue permanent and stable employment in the United States, creating uncertainty about their financial stability and general life prospects. Some federal policies may not have clear guidance directed at colleges and universities and may require additional deliberation to identify the impact on students. Counseling services, resources, and legal assistance can reassure students and mitigate the negative impact caused by rapidly changing policies and regulations that remain uncertain in terms of their duration and continuation.

Student-Athletes

Approximately 460,000 student-athletes are enrolled in U.S. colleges and universities (NCAA, 2020). Overall, student-athletes demonstrate excellence in academics with 8 out of 10 student-athletes earning a bachelor's degree (NCAA, 2020). The daily life of the student-athlete is distinct from the other students given the specific time demands of their training and competition program. Student-athletes must balance their time between academics and athletics, and they may have limited availability to build social connections beyond the athletic program as a result of their tightly packed schedule. As colleges and universities seek to support student-athletes, they may consider providing support services and wellbeing programs located on the athletic campus or closer to training facilities. For general wellbeing, ensuring that other student services such as cafeterias, student services, and other central services can help student-athletes have the same ability to access nutrition and logistical support as other students.

In reviews of student-athletes, the literature suggests distinct benefits related to mental health. Athletic participation is associated with lower rates of depression and correlates with higher levels of self-esteem and connection with others (Bornheimer and Gangwisch, 2009; Pluhar et al., 2019). The team environment, which can be positive and supportive, can also create negative stressors if the presence of group conflict, peer pressure, and bullying (Post and Kelley, 2018). Additionally, if the broader campus environment does not have a positive culture toward students from historically marginalized groups, student-athletes from those backgrounds may experience additional discrimination and harassment given their higher visibility on campus resulting from their role as an athlete (Post and Kelley, 2018).

Student-athletes may also face unique stressors related to athletic performance. Perfectionism is a trait common to high-performing individuals, including musicians and researchers, and student-athletes can encounter lowered mood or self-esteem after a relative change in position on the team or a poor competitive performance (Post and Kelley, 2018). In the event of injury or leaving the team, student-athletes may experience isolation from social networks, the loss of their identity, and having access withdrawn to special academic, health, and financial support. Wellbeing programs tailored for the needs of student-athletes can help build additional coping mechanisms, provide an environment to share challenges outside of the team dynamic, and offer students who are temporarily or permanently on leave from athletics support to develop an identity outside athletics. During COVID-19, the athletic seasons for many student-athletes have been suspended without certainty of return and, for some athletes, reduced or zero access to training facilities. While research specific to the wellbeing of student-athletes remains limited, the University of Michigan's Athletes Connected research aims to increase awareness of mental health issues, reduce the stigma of help-seeking, and promote positive coping skills among student-athletes overall and during the COVID-19 pandemic (Kern et al., 2016).[8] For example, in one pilot study, an educational intervention for varsity athletes that featured presentations that provided an "overview of mental health, two videos highlighting former student-athletes' struggles with mental illnesses, and a discussion at the end with the

---

[8] Additional information is available at https://athletesconnected.umich.edu (accessed September 29, 2020).

former athletes portrayed in the videos" found, through surveys of 626 student athletes, "significant increases in knowledge and positive attitudes toward mental health and help-seeking" (Kern et al., 2016).

Graduate Students

While many student services on university campuses are open to both undergraduates and graduate students, the needs of graduate students differ in terms of their socioemotional development, life expectations, professional demands, and academic stressors. As noted in the National Academies' *Graduate STEM Education for the 21st Century*, "High-pressure environments, cloudy career prospects, an imbalance of work and life, and leadership style of one's advisor also contribute to health problems or unhealthy mental status of graduate students."(NASEM, 2018a, p. 83). The ongoing efforts of the Council of Graduate Schools' Graduate Student Mental Health and Well-being Initiative[9] pays increased attention to the needs of graduate students. Launched in August 2019 in partnership with the Jed Foundation, the two-year initiative will examine the barriers related to care for graduate students and review the evidence-base for practices (Hazelrigg and Woodworth, 2019). The COVID pandemic and accompanying economic crisis have exacerbated pressures on graduate students as job prospects have become even more ambiguous than they were before since so many institutions are cutting back on staffing and the like.

Undergraduate students typically have general education requirements mandating a broad exploration of campus, extracurricular activities, and residential life. As a result, undergraduates often traverse a larger area on campus than master's and doctoral students, who may be enrolled in a specific program located in a handful of buildings, spend more time off campus, and may be located in another location for field research. Programs and services may be in buildings that primarily serve undergraduates or in areas of the campus that are unknown to graduate students. For graduate students who also have teaching assistantships, location of services can matter in that a graduate student may not want to seek support in the same location where they may encounter their undergraduate students or mentees. For students who have relocated for field research or to complete their dissertation in another city, virtual programs, and services, including telehealth or other distance health options, can provide alternatives to in-person sessions.

Educational demands and professional development may cause stress to graduate students, notably if the existing academic, career, and wellbeing resources on campus feel geared to an undergraduate audience. As academic research funding and tenure-track faculty positions have become more difficult to secure, graduate

---

[9] Dr. Daniel Eisenberg served on the National Academies committee on mental health, substance use, and wellbeing and the Council of Graduate Schools Graduate Student Mental Health and Well-being Initiative. Dr. Susanna Harris, a consultant for the National Academies, served on the CGS Initiative.

students who have invested significant time in their life pursuing that career may experience a loss of identity that is distinct for students at that stage of their careers. As a result, they may require help both seeking a job in a nonacademic setting and dealing with the disappointment of not achieving what for many graduate students is a life-time goal (Iarovici and Alexander, 2018).

Students experiencing these stressors can benefit from career advisors and wellbeing services that acknowledge this critical shift in identity and have knowledge of the job market for graduate students. While many of these stressors may align with the normative growth and development issues common to young adults, graduate programs may benefit from providing specialized support services that allow students to build stress management and coping mechanisms that will benefit them throughout their studies and into future roles.

Loneliness, isolation, and competition can also have a noted presence in the life of a graduate student (Ray et al., 2019). Unlike undergraduate students, graduate students often do not participate in introduction to campus programs and do not learn about various supports available to them, and they often have fewer opportunities to join extracurricular activities and build support networks. Graduate programs may be small and isolated from other departments, which can limit the development of friendships and social relationships that can help students create a sense of belonging. In departments and programs where competition for grants, papers, or general status is the norm, the environment can turn students away from each other. Without bridges to a broader community, students may experience isolation, loneliness, and lack a social system that can help individuals cope with their struggles.

For students who have strong social networks at home, leaving an established social structure can also create separation as families and friends may not understand the nature of graduate work. Additionally, graduate students may also experience financial stress if they compare their stipends to peers who work full time and receive salaries (Iarovici and Alexander, 2018). As mentioned previously, students who are completing research or field assignments may also lack the social infrastructure of both their home environment and program, and, depending on the location, may not have reliable means of communicating with those to whom they are close and from whom they can get support.

As with student-athletes, graduate students often demand perfection from themselves and internalize high expectations (Iarovici and Alexander, 2018). One phenomenon common to graduate students in high-pressure, competitive programs is imposter syndrome. The term was coined to describe a trend observed in women in which they believe they are not as competent and skilled as everyone thinks they are despite outstanding academic and professional accomplishments (Clance and Imes, 1978). This phenomenon is also not uncommon in graduate students, many of whom may discount their hard-earned achievements such as admissions, publishing a paper, or getting accepted into a conference while they attribute any setbacks to personal failings (NASEM, 2020). Graduate students who belong to groups that have been historically excluded in their discipline and program or who are in programs that have not created an inclusive environment can feel additional scrutiny (NASEM, 2018a). Given the siloed nature of graduate programs, wellbeing programs and community services that help link students to others who share similar backgrounds, transdisciplinary research interests, extracurricular activities, or interest in issues on campus can give students who may not feel belonging in their program the chance to create a social system with peers.

Graduate students may be exposed to social and professional arenas as they begin to attend conferences and build relationships outside of their program or institution with an eye toward their future careers. Events such as conferences, workshops, and seminars may include a level of professional decorum and protocol to which they have not been exposed previously. Learning how to navigate these settings can cause additional stress, uncertainty, and lack of belonging. These issues may be particularly felt by students who are BIPOC and or hold other historically excluded identities and who experience feelings of isolation in their program and even their field in the event there are limited students and faculty with similar identities.

Graduate students may also feel a lack of control and agency related to their relationship with a research advisor. While the apprenticeship model that often exists between the researcher and the student may go well, the dyadic structure and its inherent power differential pose risks in the event conflict occurs (NASEM, 2018a). There have been efforts to diffuse the power differential by offering graduate students the ability to have multiple mentors and providing networking events to expand a students' pool of mentors and advocates. Lab rotations to test research interests (in applicable fields) and policies to mediate and ease conflict between students and their advisors can also help reduce the adverse effects of a power differential. For some disciplines, the stigma around pursuing careers outside of academia remain, and students may feel pressure to conform to the tenure-track career path. Providing students with other ways to explore careers through seminars, internships, workshops, alumni networks, and graduate-specific professional advisors can help alleviate the burden on research advisors and provide students a place to learn without stigma.

In 2019, the National Academies released a study with evidence-based findings and recommendations related to the science of mentorship in science, technology, engineering, mathematics, and medicine. While this report, *The Science of Effective Mentorship in STEMM*, did not focus on mental health specifically, the report does note how mentoring can impact student development and wellbeing and the importance of identity in mentoring relationships. The report notes the benefits of a positive mentoring relationship for undergraduate and graduate students and discusses some of the negative consequences of a poor relationship. Undergraduate students who participate in mentored research experiences are more likely to stay in STEMM, and students who perceive their mentors as effective are more likely to pursue doctoral programs in related fields. Graduate students who perceive their mentors as effective are more likely to persist in academic decisions and publish research than students who are not mentored (NASEM, 2019b). For all students, the report references the need to build cross-cultural competencies in mentors to avoid causing harm related to a mentee's identity. Mentor relationships that do not include respect for mentee identity correlate with depression, reduced psychological wellbeing, and lower academic or professional performance (NASEM, 2019b).

While undergraduate students benefit from positive mentorship interactions, graduate students and postdoctoral researchers often have multiple mentors, each serving a different function, such as research advisor, or career advisor. Graduate students and postdoctoral researchers may often feel dependent on a primary research advisor for feedback on their research, funding, and connections to the field.

Overall, the research on wellbeing and mental health for graduate students remains limited in comparison to undergraduate students. As is true with the other groups discussed in this chapter, graduate students are not a monolithic group, and their identities also intersect with others in this chapter. Effective support for graduate students would benefit from increased research and program evaluation. See Chapter 6 on the Research Agenda for details on recommended research.

Medical Students

The medical profession has come under scrutiny for a work culture that is exceedingly demanding and can push practitioners beyond their tolerance limits and lead to "burnout" and a range of mental health issues. While this section highlights the mental health issues of medical students, it is important to note that other health professionals face similar challenges, and thus, the discussion likely applies more broadly to these professions and the students studying in these fields. Professional societies from the Association of American Medical Colleges (AAMC), the National Academy of Medicine, and the American Medical Association have conducted research on the toll burnout can take on the medical profession where approximately half of physicians report burnout symptoms: "Burnout is a syndrome characterized by a high degree of emotional exhaustion and depersonalization (i.e., cynicism), and a low sense of personal accomplishment at work" (NASEM, 2019c). As a result of inconsistent definitions, the overall body of research on burnout in academic medicine should be reviewed with caution.

Medical students and other health professionals have a distinct educational trajectory and encounter significant stressors throughout their training. An international meta-analysis found that the prevalence of self-reported depression in medical students to be 27.2 percent, but only 15.7 percent of students with positive screens for depression went on to seek mental health treatment (Iarovici and Alexander, 2018). Substance use by medical students and trainees has also been documented at higher rates; data showed that 91.3 percent and 26.2 percent of medical students consumed alcohol and used marijuana, respectively, and that additional studies on patterns of substance use are needed to prevent substance use disorders among medical students (Ayala et al., 2017). The gap between positive screens and the decision to pursue treatment has deeper implications—an alarming increase in suicidal thoughts. One large meta-analysis found that over 10 percent of medical students have had suicidal thinking over the past 12 months (Iarovici and Alexander, 2018). Other studies have examined the prevalence of mental health disorders among medical students (Guille et al., 2010; Rotenstein et al., 2016; Sen et al., 2010).

As with student-athletes and graduate students, students in most health care professions operate in a highly competitive environment with demanding expectations on performance and hours dedicated to developing practice. The long hours can lead to reduced sleep, limited physical activity, separation from important relationships, strain on nutrition, and isolation from interaction outside of the cohort and the training environment. The demands and expectations of medical school and other health care training programs may leave students feeling that they do not have time in their schedules to seek additional services. As mentioned previously, the drive for perfectionism can push students to internalize stress and feel that revealing mental health challenges would make them less qualified for medical practice. Providing wellbeing programs that help individuals retain healthy life habits, workshops that focus on reducing stigma around seeking mental health services, and policies that protect students from overwork can provide students with multiple levels to seek assistance. Additionally, there is some research to support the idea that changes to curriculum and grading practices in medical school may reduce stress (Bloodgood et al., 2009; Slavin et al., 2014; Slavin and Chibnall, 2016; Slavin et al., 2014), for example, noted that "efficient changes to course content, contact hours, scheduling, grading, electives, learning communities, and required resilience/mindfulness experiences were associated with significantly lower levels of depression symptoms, anxiety symptoms, and stress, and significantly higher levels of community cohesion, in medical students."

Students in health care professions often operate in an environment separate from the rest of a university's main campus, so the health affairs campus has an important leadership role in shaping education and work settings. The medical education system particularly has strong roots in the apprenticeship model and has been identified as more hierarchical. This can be characterized as a system where trainees feel more responsible for following direction from their supervisors than other disciplines, and the culture is less supportive of questions or pushing back against figures of authority (Martinez et al., 2014). To understand the challenges that clinicians in health care face, the National Academy of Medicine has created a conceptual framework of factors that impact clinician wellbeing and resilience across all health professions, specialties, settings, and career stages (see Figure 3-1).

FACTORS AFFECTING CLINICIAN WELL-BEING AND RESILIENCE

This conceptual model depicts the factors associated with clinician well-being and resilience; applies these factors across all health care professions, specialties, settings, and career stages; and emphasizes the link between clinician well-being and outcomes for clinicians, patients, and the health system. The model should be used to understand well-being, rather than as a diagnostic or assessment tool. In electronic form, the external and individual factors of the conceptual model are hyperlinked to corresponding landing pages on the Clinician Well-Being Knowledge Hub. The Clinician Well-Being Knowledge Hub provides additional information and resources. The conceptual model will be revised as the field develops and more information becomes available.

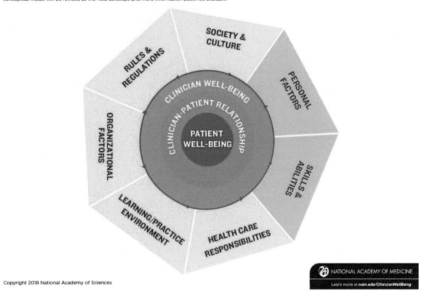

Copyright 2018 National Academy of Sciences

NATIONAL ACADEMY OF MEDICINE
Learn more at *nam.edu/ClinicianWellBeing*

FIGURE 3-1 Factors affecting clinician wellbeing and resilience.
Source: NASEM, 2019c.

The full tool[10] provides lists of components for each of the external and internal factors (the yellow and blue units on the outside of the model). Given that the medical training environment has a history of hierarchy and dominance from leadership, schools and departments that review and address wellbeing can help shift the climate for medical students and trainees as well.

Neurodiverse Students

While some students with developmental disorders, such as autism spectrum disorder (ASD) or cognitive and learning disabilities, may identify as students with disability, there has been a movement toward thinking about these students under the concept of neurodiversity. In the early 1990s, researchers coined the term as part of a civil rights movement for individuals with neurologically based disabilities (Armstrong, 2017). These investigators worked to shift the paradigm

---

[10] The full tool is available online at https://nam.edu/clinicianwellbeing/resources/factors-affecting-clinician-well-being-and-resilience-conceptual-model.

from a deficit-oriented model, which frames these individuals as operating with an impaired sense of cognitive and emotional properties, to a strength-based model where "neurological differences are to be recognized and respected as any other human variation" (Masataka, 2018). While the movement originated with ASD activism, the umbrella for neurodiversity has expanded to include learning disabilities, ADD/ADHD, intellectual disability, and social and emotional disorders (Armstrong, 2017).

Developments in screening, treatment, and support for neurodiverse individuals in their childhood and adolescence has increased their ability to prepare for the academic and psychosocial demands of higher education. Some campuses have developed specific programs designed to support neurodiverse students, including the College of William and Mary's Neurodiversity Initiative and the London School of Economics' Dyslexia and Neurodiversity program (Armstrong, 2017). For other colleges and universities, accommodations for students with learning disabilities must comply with ADA (see Chapter 4 and the section on *Federal Regulations for Higher Education* for more information on the Americans with Disabilities Act). Additional research on neurodiverse students in higher education is needed to determine the efficacy of policies and practices intended to support their wellbeing and academic achievement (see Chapter 6 on the Research Agenda).

Post-Traditional or Non-Traditional Students

Colleges and universities were originally designed to educate white men whose families could afford to support additional years of education in a residential setting. The legacy of these early undergraduates has persisted, living on in the stereotype of a college student in their late teens to early twenties, often living on or near campus. As noted in Chapter 2, there has been a growing number of students who enroll in higher education as older adults or who return to campus to seek additional credentials. The National Center for Education Statistics projected that 38 percent of the almost 20 million students enrolled in institutions of higher education would be 25 years and older—so-called post-traditional learners—in 2018 (Bruce-Sanford and Soares, 2019).

For colleges and universities, many post-traditional students have a different set of issues than first-time, full-time residential college student attending out of the K-12 system. These individuals are more likely to have long-term partners or spouses and other dependents, be employed full time, and be veterans (Iarovici, 2014). With these different life circumstances, post-traditional students are more likely to have other responsibilities and seek support in other ways, such as needing to find childcare and have flexible scheduling (Iarovici, 2014; McBride, 2019). Post-traditional students may have schedules that limit their ability to attend on-site wellbeing programs or to make appointments with counseling services.

For some students, asynchronous resources or virtual services they can access from home, might be more accessible, notably for students enrolled in online or hybrid programs who do not regularly come to the physical campus. Providing extended hours in evenings and weekends, additional locations, and connections to community providers who may be closer to the student's residence or employer can help students with access as well. While not all post-traditional students attend community college, it is more likely that community college students have challenges accessing basic life needs such as housing, food, transportation, and stable access to technology often considered essential to higher education, such as computers and wi-fi. For students who are caregivers, these needs can compound as they may serve as a primary provider. While these issues may be concentrated at community colleges, they are not limited to them. Colleges and universities that support students' basic needs can mitigate some life stressors, and enhance wellbeing for those students, and these services have been shown to correlate to higher academic outcomes such as retention and completion.

Access to additional services and extended hours can make programs and support more accessible to post-traditional students, but the research on the mental health and wellbeing of these students remains limited (Cadigan et al., 2020; Iarovici, 2014). Some research has focused on understanding the motivations for post-traditional students, which can help staff and faculty set expectations and work with students toward their goals. As many post-traditional students seek education to advance their careers, their efforts and performance may look different than traditional students. Research has shown that older students may be adversely affected by the emphasis on grades or other extrinsic factors. Better outcomes for older students can be achieved by validating their academic performance and autonomy and treating them as active partners in learning (Iarovici, 2014).

For post-traditional students in academic programs with mostly traditional students, there may be other ways to help students feel a sense of belonging. Post-traditional students, who are more likely to have additional demands with work and family, may not be able to attend office hours, group meetings, or access programs and services. They may feel isolated from the other students because of differences in life stage and have a reduced ability to develop bonds through extracurricular and social activities. Given the additional demands associated with the lives of post-traditional students and their presence in community college, centralized student counseling centers can provide greater ease of access to students and can improve academic outcomes such as retention, transfer, and graduation (Van Brunt and ACCA PAPA Committee, 2010). As noted in previous sections, loneliness and isolation can make students of any age and life situation feel less welcome, which can adversely affect an individual's wellbeing (Iarovici, 2014).

Sexual and Gender Minorities

Sexual and gender minority (SGM) is a term that has developed to encompass the full range of identities related to sexual orientation and gender. The National Institute of Health's Sexual and Gender and Minority Research Office defines SGM populations as including, but not limited to,

> "...individuals who identify as lesbian, gay, bisexual, asexual, transgender, two-spirit, queer, and/or intersex. Individuals with same-sex or -gender attractions or behaviors and those with a difference in sex development are included, too. These populations also encompass those who do not self-identify with one of these terms but whose sexual orientation, gender identity or expression, or reproductive development is characterized by non-binary constructs of sexual orientation, gender, and/or sex" (SGMRO, 2020).

For the purposes of this report, SGM also encompasses identities that have been considered under LGBTQIAP+, which include individuals who are questioning, pansexual, or polyamorous. In the 2019 ACHA-NCHA fall survey, 17.9 percent of undergraduate and graduate students described their sexual orientation in categories other than straight/heterosexual.[11] For gender identity, 1.2 percent of students identified outside of the binary woman/female and man/male categories, and 1.8 percent responded as transgendered. As with other populations, students in this category are not monolithic and their identities may shift during their time on campus. For some identities that may comprise a small proportion of the total, recognition of their sexual and gender identities is critical to recognize the full humanity of these students and combat stigma associated with SGM identities.

---

[11] The other options available for students includes asexual (0.7 percent); bisexual (8.8 percent); gay (2.0 percent); lesbian (1.3 percent); pansexual (1.6 percent); queer (1.2 percent); questioning (1.9 percent); and identity not listed above (0.4 percent). The total will not amount to 100 percent, as there were also invalid responses and non-responses.

Note from the ACHA-NCHA survey on the use of sex and gender: Survey responses are reported by sex based on the responses to questions 67A, 67B, and 67C. For the purpose of the ACHA-NCHA report documents, respondents are reported as male or female only when their responses to these three questions are consistent with one another. If gender identity is consistent with sex at birth AND "no" is selected for transgender, then respondents are designated as either male or female. If respondents select "yes" for transgender OR their sex at birth is not consistent with their gender identity, then they are designated as non-binary. A respondent that selects "intersex" for sex at birth, "no" for transgender, and man or woman for gender identity are designated as male or female. A respondent that selects "intersex" for sex at birth, "yes" for transgender, or selects a gender identity other than man or woman are designated as non-binary. A respondent that skips any of the three questions is designated as unknown. Only three of the four categories are displayed in this report. Respondents categorized as non-binary are included in the Total column but are not presented in a separate column. When the total of any given row is higher than the sum of the male, female, and unknown respondents, the difference can be attributed to non-binary respondents that selected the response option presented in that row.

For many individuals, their time on campus may parallel a developmental and life stage where they explore sexual and gender identity. Some students may not have felt comfortable working through this aspect of their selves if they lived in a hostile community, while other students may not have developed or recognized a desire to investigate until they arrive at their college or university. Peer support groups that focus on SGM issues can help students who are in the process of exploring their identity, experiencing challenges in close relationships, or validating their identity. Other efforts through residential life and student services that recognize SGM students, provide guidance and training for friends and allies, and offer informal ways to seek help for students in distress or facing harassment based on their SGM identity can help reduce bias and make students feel more welcome.

Wellbeing and mental health support for SGM students should incorporate inclusive methods that recognize the legacy of harm embedded in the history of U.S. laws, medicine, and society. For SGM individuals who choose to enter therapy, other fears may arise such as a concern about information being discovered outside of the sessions, hospitalization, limited resources for those with a SGM identity, and lack of health professionals with experience in working with issues common in the SGM community (Shah, Eshel, and McGlynn, 2018). For colleges and universities seeking to support students, having health professionals who practice inclusive approaches that make strong efforts to normalize minority gender identities and sexualities and who become well versed in the nuances of the SGM culture and vernacular can limit the impact of anti-SGM stigma on mental health (Shah, Eshel, and McGlynn, 2018).

Currently, there is limited research regarding approaches that are effective in supporting SGM students.[12] As the research base continues to grow, there are ways that health professionals, as well as staff, faculty, students, and others on campus, can develop inclusive practices. One example is the use of gender expansive language that goes beyond the gender binary of she/hers and he/his to include the singular they/their or the use of the honorific to "Mx." Affirming students' gender through pronouns without qualification (e.g., "preferred pronouns") is described by the Human Rights Campaign as a way to support others (HRCF, 2018). Introductions in settings across campus, notably those led by individuals in a position of authority (e.g., faculty, staff, administrators, and student leaders) that include the option to include pronouns can normalize non-binary pronoun

---

[12] The Committee on Population of the National Academies of Sciences, Engineering, and Medicine will undertake a consensus study that will review the available data and future research needs on persons of diverse sexualities and genders (e.g., Lesbian, Gay, Bisexual, Transgender, Queer/Questioning, Plus/LGBTQ+ and Men who have Sex with Men/MSM). It will also include persons with differences in sex development (sometimes known as intersex), along multiple intersecting dimensions across the life course. The report is due for release in late 2020 or early 2021.

use and allow students to share that identity with others.[13] This may be repeated over time with new individuals and to allow students to express updated pronouns if they have changes.

Within the student population with SGM identities, colleges and universities may seek additional guidance related to appropriate treatment of transgender individuals. In comparison to cisgender peers, transgender youth aged 12-18 years report higher rates of experiences associated with negative health outcomes including "violence, victimization, substance use, and suicide risk, and, although more likely to report some sexual risk behaviors, were also more likely to be tested for human immunodeficiency virus (HIV) infection" (Johns et al., 2019). Wellbeing services and counselors can develop an awareness of these issues as a context for the fears transgender and transitioning students may express. Mental health services can also support transgender and students in transition by having a working knowledge of the campus resources and even administrative processes such as the ability to change names and pronouns in university systems and serve as a "guide [in the] gender exploration process or to obtain a support letter for therapy with hormones or surgery; or for reasons completely unrelated to gender, such as relationship issues or anxiety" (Khan and Hansen, 2018).

Transgender students and students who do not identify along the female/ male binary face harm when forced to reply to government surveys, school paperwork, and other indices that do not list their identity as an option. Additionally, transgender students who have transitioned and have chosen a new name face the risk of being "deadnamed," the use of their birth or given name, in medical or administrative settings if they have not had a legal name change. The Human Rights Campaign 2018 Youth Report describes better outcomes for students, such as decreased instances of anxiety and depression, when they feel supported by their environment (HRCF, 2018). For example, providing administrative options to allow students to list their names and pronouns, even if a legal name and sex assigned at birth are also required, can affirm student identities, provide faculty and staff with accurate information about the student, and reduce harm.

Student Survivors of Trauma

Consistent with national data in the general population, the student body of most every college and university is likely to include individuals who arrive to campus with a history of trauma (Arnekrans et al., 2018; Davidson, 2017). One important metric of trauma and adversity is the landmark public health study on Adverse Childhood Experiences (ACE), which includes experiences of individuals from birth to 18 years old of abuse and neglect of all kinds as well as parental mental illness, substance use, divorce, incarceration, and domestic violence,

---

[13] The option to share pronouns gives students the opportunity to opt-out if they do not feel comfortable sharing. Mandatory sharing can cause students who are exploring gender pronoun use distress.

showing lifelong impacts on physical development, mental health, and risk taking (Felitti et al., 1998).[14] In 2016, 34 million children under 18, or nearly 50 percent of all U.S. children, experienced one ACE and greater than 20 percent had experienced two or more (CAMHI, 2018). While there is more research on trauma-informed educational approaches for children under 18 and for the K-12 system, there has been increasing attention to understanding trauma's impact on postsecondary learners and creating strategies for the higher education setting (Plimb, Bush, and Kersevich, 2016). Because of cognitive, self-regulatory, and interpersonal challenges that often result from histories of trauma, research increasingly indicates a correlation between ACE or trauma and lowered educational attainment (Metzler et al., 2017). Existing research regarding the link between developmental trauma and academic resilience, persistence, and completion in college students indicates that the dynamics between trauma and academic outcomes are complex, not well understood, and in need of further research (Anders, Frasier, and Shallcross, 2012; Arnekrans et al., 2018; Baker et al., 2016; Duncan, 2000; Hardner, Wolf, and Rinfrette, 2018; Hinojosa et al., 2019; Metzler et al., 2017; Read et al., 2012).

Certain student groups have a greater likelihood of exposure to trauma, including women, individuals from the SGM community, students with disabilities, and students who are BIPOC (Anders, Frasier, and Shallcross, 2012; Austin, Herrick, and Proescholdbell, 2015; Edman, Watson, and Patron, 2016; Read et al., 2011; Slopen et al., 2016). In addition, whether they have experienced previous trauma or not, students may encounter traumatic events during their time as a student. Research on exposure to a potentially traumatizing event (PTE) during higher education remains limited. There are also time periods that correlate with higher rates of PTE exposure, with up to 50 percent of college students reporting a PTE in their first year (Davidson, 2017).

Sexual harassment and assault constitute a specific form of trauma that has received increased attention in past years. The 2018 National Academies report *Sexual Harassment of Women: Climate, Culture, and Consequences in Academic Sciences, Engineering, and Medicine* (NASEM, 2018b) states the prevalence of sexual harassment as a key finding.[15] Not only is sexual harassment a common event, it is also one that those who have been sexually harassed tend to experience

---

[14] The National Survey of Children's Health ACE's 2016 assessed exposure to the following nine experiences: (1) Somewhat often/very often hard to get by on income; (2) Parent/guardian divorced or separated; (3) Parent/guardian died; (4) Parent/guardian served time in jail; (5) Saw or heard violence in the home; (6) Victim/witness of neighborhood violence; (7) Lived with anyone mentally ill, suicidal, or depressed; (8) Lived with anyone with alcohol or drug problem; and (9) Often treated or judged unfairly due to race/ethnicity (CAMHI, 2018). See: https://www.cahmi.org/wp-content/uploads/2018/05/aces_fact_sheet.pdf.

[15] While sexual harassment is experienced by people of all genders, the scope of this report focused on the sexual harassment of women specifically. While this report focused primarily on sciences, engineering, and medicine, it referenced data and research from other areas. Unlike this report, *Sexual Harassment of Women* looked at women at all roles in academia, not students specifically.

more than once. In a 2016 study of female graduate students that self-reported experiencing sexually harassing behavior, only one-third reported that they experienced a single incident. For women who are BIPOC and SGM women, the report notes that issues of sexual- and gender-based harassment intersect with other biases that stem from their race, ethnicity, and other identities and that sexual harassment is experienced differently (NASEM, 2018b). While the report does not specify research on the experience of SGM students, a study of employees in higher education found that SGM individuals of all genders reported higher rates of gender harassment (73 percent) and sexual harassment (40 percent) compared to heterosexual peers (30 percent and 15.5 percent, respectively) (NASEM, 2018b).

The report also includes data on the perpetrators of sexual harassment, which can provide additional information to guide prevention, as well as information of the impact of sexual harassment on the broader community. The report notes that while people of all genders experience sexual harassment, the predominant harassers are male, with 86 percent of female graduate students who experience sexual harassment from faculty or staff reporting that the harasser was male. Men are also more likely to be the perpetrators of sexually harassing behavior of other men (NASEM, 2018b). Sexual harassment does not only harm those who are targeted, as workplace research indicates that indirect exposure or the perceived level of sexual harassment in a workgroup also leads to similar negative issues as those suffered by individuals with direct experience. The presence of sexual harassment can cause trauma, create an environment that does not support wellbeing, and make individuals feel unwelcomed and more likely to leave that environment. As colleges and universities think about ways to ensure safety and wellbeing, the prevention of sexual harassment and the creation of an accountable, transparent system for addressing harassment cases can aid in those efforts.

Traumatic experiences, regardless of when they occurred, can have lifelong impacts on students. ACHA (2016) states that trauma-informed approaches "emphasize physical, psychological, and emotional safety for both providers and victims/survivors, which allows victims/survivors to rebuild a sense of safety, control, and empowerment." As campuses build trauma-informed services or adopt trauma-informed practices, it is important to remember how students might encounter different kinds of trauma. In addition to the groups previously mentioned as having a higher likelihood of trauma exposure, international students, students without documentation, and veterans may have exposure to distinct types of trauma based on their background. Colleges and universities can expand the use of a trauma-informed lens beyond programs and services for students, with trauma-informed approaches involving vigilance in anticipating and avoiding institutional practices and processes that are likely to re-traumatize individuals. Trauma-informed approaches allow services to be delivered in a way that facilitates the victim's/survivor's participation (ACHA, 2016).

The Department of Health and Human Services (2014) identified trauma-informed principles, including safety; trustworthiness and transparency; peer support; collaboration and mutuality; empowerment; and cultural, historical, and gender issues.

Student Military Service Members and Veterans

Since World War II, many veterans of the U.S. armed forces have pursued higher education after the conclusion of their service. According to the Student Veteran Association, over a million veterans have returned home since 2008 to pursue a postsecondary degree or certificate using Veterans Affairs education benefits (SVA, 2020). The student veteran population is distinct from the general population: those who served in the armed services tend to be predominately male, entered the military after high school, and are more likely to be from rural communities or the southern United States (Lauff, Chen, and Morgan, 2018). In terms of race and ethnicity, the representation of white and Black groups approximates their presence in the general population, while Asians are underrepresented, and Native Hawaiian and Pacific Islanders are overrepresented (Lauff, Chen, and Morgan, 2018). The distinctions for student service members and veterans (SSM/V) goes beyond demographic information as well in that they are adult learners who often have social, cognitive, physical, and psychological readjustment challenges when transitioning to college environments. In addition, SSM/V students can encounter unique informational and bureaucratic hurdles related to reenrolling and supporting their postsecondary education (Aikins et al., 2015).

SSM/Vs, who are likely to attend postsecondary education after service, experience many of the challenges that post-traditional and non-traditional students experience. They may feel more isolation and distance from the other students, who are likely younger, and SSM/Vs may find a challenge in adjusting to the relatively loose schedule on campus compared to the structured life in the military (Aikins et al., 2015). While many colleges and universities provide specific resources for veterans to navigate the academic, financial, and health and wellbeing services on campus, the support provided varies considerably from campus to campus. One survey found that 57 percent of 723 institutions of higher education provide programs and services specifically designed for service members, with a greater percentage of public four- and two-year colleges having veteran-specific programs than private institutions (Aikins et al., 2015). As SSM/Vs have a number of identities and may seek support through a number of campus services, online directories and resources that inform students, as well as faculty and staff who may be asked for guidance, of which services are available and where can help students navigate the full range of available support.

In addition to the challenges many veterans face in navigating higher education, there are also specific health issues, such as auditory problems, post-traumatic stress disorder (PTSD), and traumatic brain injury (TBI), that have a higher occurrence in veterans and can affect their ability to learn. These conditions, particularly when co-occurring with mental health problems, can seriously impair social and occupational functioning, including academic performance (Kuhn and McCaslin, 2018).

The impact on cognitive function and the development of learning disabilities can make SSM/Vs eligible for additional accommodations under ADA. These issues may also arise related to concussions and TBI. Of groups in higher education, SSM/Vs and student-athletes have the greatest likelihood of experiencing a TBI, most frequently a mild TBI in the form of a concussion. While there are the immediate cognitive effects of a concussion, there are also associations with repetitive injury—slower recovery and chronically-elevated post-concussive symptoms—and there are concerns that repetitive head injuries "may be associated with an increased risk of chronic neurologic, neuropsychiatric, and neurobehavioral problems, including the possibility of chronic traumatic encephalopathy" (Broglio et al., 2017). General population research has also yielded preliminary connections between repetitive injury and the development of mental health issues, including PTSD (Howlett and Stein, 2016).

More research specific to SSM/Vs (and college athletes) would provide additional guidance to colleges and universities regarding prevention, recognition, treatment, and long-term rehabilitations. Governing bodies, such as the branches of the military and the NCAA, can also use available evidence and research to shift policies to protect SSM/Vs and student-athletes. As individuals and their physicians assess cognitive capacity after a head injury, guidance about accommodations for cognitive impairment and learning disabilities can give students the additional support needed to complete coursework as well as additional mental health treatment and counseling to help with recovery. Offices that provide specific support to veterans and athletes may create resources specifically for students recovering from head injuries and those continuing to manage cognitive symptoms.

4

Clinical Mental Health and Substance Use Services for Students in Higher Education

Many colleges and universities provide services to students in a clinical setting in addition to programs focusing on general student wellbeing. These services may include general health, as well as those for students experiencing mental health and substance use problems. However, there is considerable variation in the scope of services, the level of education and professional licensure of the clinical staff, the availability of clinical providers, and the training that the providers have received to work with specific populations of students. Because use of mental health services is to be held confidential by a range of state and federal laws (e.g., the Health Insurance Portability and Accountability Act), it can be challenging for institutions to balance collaborating services across the whole student while also respecting a student's state/federal right to privacy.

In general, on-campus treatment centers and their staff are uniquely positioned, trained, and professionally focused to effectively navigate this important balancing act (e.g., working with residence life and student conduct units to proactively manage a perceived behavioral threat with mental health concerns). Depending on the size and financial resources of a campus, connections to independent, off-campus providers may also be an important part of the network of care for student mental health. Challenges exist, however, with referrals to private off-campus providers. In general, they are explicitly focused on the treatment of the individual and have considerably less training and dedicated time to overcome legal privacy concerns in order to coordinate with multiple on-campus offices. Other challenges can include distance from campus and students' lack of transportation; difficulty navigating private health insurance systems; limited coverage for mental health on many insurance plans; students' lack of health insurance generally; costs of coverage and copays; and lack of community providers or limited providers that support college students. For students able to navigate and access mental health care in the community, issues may also arise in terms of releasing information from campus providers, receipt of records back to the college or university system (such as for accommodations for learning disabilities), and continuity of care if the student leaves for vacations, field work, an internship, or another off-campus experience.

Student access to these services differs as well. The students who use these services range from those with preexisting conditions looking for support and management to students developing issues during their enrollment. There may be limitations for students in terms of availability of services (how many sessions are provided or how quickly students can be seen), times when services can be accessed, and concern about cost (even if the services are covered by student fees). Stigma may also inhibit student use of needed services. While some students may feel willing to attend a student seminar focused on wellbeing with peers or to join a department workshop focused on building a work/life balance, the stigma around mental health and substance use may also be a barrier to seeking needed services. In addition, some clinical services may require referrals for access to a psychiatrist, be required to do additional intake forms, or go on a waiting list.

This chapter discusses some of the ways in which colleges and universities are providing mental health and substance use services, beyond the wellness programs addressed in Chapter 3. It also describes the various policies that govern how higher education provides services, such as mandated alcohol and substance use education.

THE HISTORICAL AND POLICY CONTEXT FOR MENTAL HEALTH AND SUBSTANCE USE SERVICES IN HIGHER EDUCATION

The history of student health care on campuses began at Amherst College in 1861, although mental health services were not offered until the establishment of a practice at Princeton University in 1910 (Kraft, 2011). Though the American Student Health Association included "mental hygiene" as a priority in 1920, it was not until 1957 that the American College Health Association formed a section for mental health professionals and for mental health and counseling services to become a more standard feature on campuses (Kraft, 2011). Until the 1960s, U.S. colleges and universities operated *in loco parentis*, meaning they had the authority and responsibility to oversee students' personal lives and individual actions without due process (Lee, 2011).

After World War II and the increase of veterans using G.I. Bill benefits to pursue higher education, college and university enrollments increased alongside the demand for mental health professionals (Kraft, 2011).[1] At this time, mental health services were divided between psychiatric consultation and student health in one unit and counseling centers in another. While funding for counseling centers originally came from general institutional revenue, restructuring occurred when colleges and universities began to charge separate fees to cover health services.[2] As campuses looked to streamline counseling services and shift costs for mental health counseling to student health fees and/or separate health insurance coverage, many schools merged counseling services with psychiatric and mental health services. As Kraft (2011) notes "the multidisciplinary mental health service became the norm on campuses rather than the exception." In 1950, the Association of University and College Counseling Center Directors (AUCCCD) was founded to create a community of mental health leaders in higher education. Today, AUCCCD represents nearly 1,000 college and university counseling centers. The American College Counseling Association (ACCA), American Psychological Association, and American College Health Association also have sections and program devoted to student mental health.

Federal Regulations for Higher Education

Americans with Disabilities Act

In 1990, Congress passed the Americans with Disabilities Act (ADA) to protect the civil rights of individuals with disabilities related to employment, public services, and places of public use. Similar to laws passed to protect individuals from discrimination based on race, religion, sex, and national origin, the ADA's goal is to "assure equal opportunity, full participation, independent living, and economic self-sufficiency for Americans with Disabilities" (ADA National Network, 2020).

The ADA includes provisions for access and participation in postsecondary education. U.S. legislation has included policies regarding support to transition from K-12 to higher education; efforts by disability services offices at universities to improve student access; principles of universal design and accommodations to ensure accessibility; and a growing emphasis on the use of technology and diversity within the student population (ADA National Network, 2020). For a student to receive protection under the ADA, they must have a "physical or mental impairment that substantially limits one or more major life activities" (e.g.,

---

[1] The G.I. Bill did not make college more accessible for all veterans: "While the introduction of generous student aid through the G.I. Bill held the promise of significantly reducing black-white gaps in educational opportunity and long-run economic outcomes, the G.I. Bill exacerbated rather than narrowed the economic and educational differences between blacks and whites among men from the South" (Turner and Bound, 2003).

[2] Information about current funding models and related challenges appear in Chapter 5 in the section Insufficient Funding.

learning, caring for oneself, walking, seeing, hearing, speaking, and working); have a record of having had this type of impairment; and be regarded as having this type of impairment (Jed Foundation, 2008).

On campus, colleges and universities must ensure that faculty, other instructors (including graduate students and postdoctoral researchers), and staff comply with the ADA in educational settings, including extracurricular activities, by extending the time for test taking or completing course work; by substituting specific courses to meet degree requirements; and by modifying test taking or performance evaluations so as not to discriminate against a person's sensory, speaking, or motor impairments, unless that is what is being tested. Accommodations can also include providing auxiliary aids and services such as qualified sign language interpreters, note takers, and readers, as well as adaptive equipment and braille, large print, and electronic formats of print materials (American Psychological Association, 2020).

Students with disorders that impact their cognitive and emotional functions, such as attention deficit disorder and attention deficit and hyperactivity disorder (ADD/ADHD) and autism spectrum disorder can receive protection under the ADA, too (see the section on Neurodiverse Students in Chapter 3). Students who are pregnant or have pregnancy-related health issues may also seek accommodations through the ADA.

Drug-Free Schools and Communities Acts and Campus Recovery Programs

In 1989, under the Drug-Free Schools and Communities Act, legislators amended the Higher Education Act by requiring colleges and universities to "invest considerable energy in implementing substance abuse prevention programs, distributing written policies, and evaluating program outcomes" (Custer and Kent, 2019). Prevention programs must meet a number of minimum federal standards for employees and students regarding unlawful possession; description of laws regarding possession and distribution at the local, state, and federal level; description of health risks associated with substance use disorders; support, treatment, and recovery programs made available; and a clear statement about disciplinary actions used against those who violate policy (DeRicco, 2006). Colleges and universities may be subject to additional state and local regulations.

Family Educational Rights and Privacy Act of 1974

The Family Educational Rights and Privacy Act (FERPA) established in 1974 to protect student educational records, applies to all schools receiving funds from the Department of Education (ED, 2020). Without a waiver, FERPA precludes colleges and universities from sharing academic records except in limited circumstances, such as when there is an urgent need to protect the health and safety of a student or another person on campus. In the event that an individual poses a risk to themselves or others, university officials are permitted but not required to inform appropriate individuals (HHS and ED, 2019). (See discussion of the Health Insurance Portability and Accountability Act of 1996 [HIPAA] below for additional information.)

Health Insurance Portability and Accountability Act of 1996

HIPAA ensures the privacy of medical records for all individuals, and it has specific implications for students. The act protects an individual's medical records by limiting electronic access to the records to health care service providers. This means that families of students cannot access their health care records without a release of information signed by the student. It also means that student mental health records (included health care and counseling) cannot be transferred electronically to others at the college or university without a signed release of information, except to a very limited set of university personnel such as police or physicians in situations where there is a risk of imminent harm (HHS and ED, 2019).

Federal Funding for Mental Health, Substance Use, and Wellbeing Research and Programs

The Garrett Lee Smith Memorial Act

In addition to funding from sources within the college or university, there have been some federal programs that have sought to intervene in college mental health (see Box 4-1). The Garrett Lee Smith Memorial Act (GLSMA, 2004) was signed into law in October 2004 and with an original authorization for $82 million in grants related to suicide prevention to be administered by the Substance Abuse and Mental Health Services Administration (SAMHSA). GLSMA provided federal funding for the first time to states, tribes, and colleges to implement community-based suicide prevention programs for youth and young adults (Godoy Garraza et al., 2018). As of 2020, GLSMA had supported 243 total State tribal grants in 50 states and the District of Columbia, 67 tribes or tribal organizations, and 309 grants to 269 institutions of higher education. Institutions of higher education have used GLSMA funds to develop comprehensive, collaborative, well-coordinated, and evidence-based approaches to (1) enhance mental health services for all college students, including those at risk for suicide, depression, serious mental illness (SMI)/serious emotional disturbances (SED), and/or substance use disorders that can lead to school failure; (2) prevent mental and substance use disorders; (3) promote help-seeking behavior and reduce negative public attitudes; and (4) improve the identification and treatment of at-risk college students so they can successfully complete their studies. It is expected that this program will reduce the adverse consequences of SMI/SED and substance use disorders, including suicidal behavior, substance-related injuries, and school failure (SAMHSA FOA SM18-003).

While students have been the primary audience for Campus GLSMA-funded efforts, gatekeeper training,[3] intended to provide suicide prevention and awareness to a broader audience, reached other groups including college faculty, college counseling and health center staff, residential life staff, campus security, parents and guardians, and primary care staff (Godoy Garraza et al., 2018).

Figure 4-1 shows various suicide prevention strategies employed by GLSMA grantees, from outreach and awareness training to traditional healing practices. Data are available at the category level for state, tribal, and campus grantees in cohorts 1-12. Data collection at the strategy level began in 2010; therefore, data are available at the strategy level for state and tribal grantees in cohorts 4-12 and campus grantees in cohorts 3-12. Table 4-1 provides details on grantee participation by level of intervention.

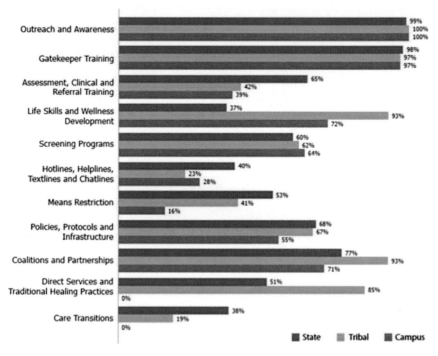

FIGURE 4-1 Grantees' utilization of various suicide prevention intervention categories. Source: SAMHSA. Prevention Strategies Inventory, June 2019, State/tribal cohorts 1-12, campus cohorts 1-12.

---

[3] Chapter 5 includes a more detailed discussion of gatekeeper training programs.

TABLE 4-1 Grantee Participation in Prevention Strategies Inventory

Level of Data	State Grantees	Tribal Grantees	Campus Grantees
Category	124 of 124	73 of 75	266 of 266
Strategy	93 of 93	66 of 68	211 of 211

Source: SAMHSA.

BOX 4-1
Federal Funding Agencies and Mental Health,
Substance Use, and Wellbeing

Several agencies in the U.S. federal government oversee funding for research and programs related to mental health, substance use, and wellbeing. Funding for colleges and universities may exist in broader programs for adolescents, young adults, or adults broadly. The federal government also collects data on health behaviors, which also can include college students; however, the data do not necessarily separate enrolled students from their age-matched peers.

National Institute on Alcohol Abuse and Alcoholism (NIAAA): NIAAA was founded in 1974, and it supports and conducts research on the impact of alcohol use on human health and wellbeing. It is the largest funder of alcohol research in the world, with a budget of $545.4 million in FY 2020. The agency does not fund direct services (https://www.niaaa.nih.gov).

National Institute for Drug Abuse (NIDA): NIDA was founded in 1974, and its mission is to advance science on the causes and consequences of drug use and addiction and to apply that knowledge to improve individual and public health. In this regard, NIDA addresses the most fundamental and essential questions about drug use—from detecting and responding to emerging drug use trends and understanding how drugs work in the brain and body, to developing and testing new approaches to treatment and prevention. NIDA had a budget of $1.42 billion in FY 2020. NIDA does not fund direct services (https://www.drugabuse.gov).

National Institute of Mental Health (NIMH): NIMH was founded in 1949, and its mission is to transform the understanding and treatment of mental illnesses through basic and clinical research, paving the way for prevention, recovery, and cure. NIMH had a budget of $1.86 billion in FY 2020. It does not fund direct services (https://www.nimh.nih.gov).

Substance Abuse and Mental Health Services Administration (SAMHSA): SAMHSA was founded in 1992, and it is the agency within the Department of Health and Human Services that leads public health efforts to advance the behavioral health of the nation. SAMHSA's mission is to reduce the impact of substance abuse and mental illness on America's communities. SAMHSA had a budget of $5.74 billion in FY 2020. It does operate grant programs to organizations that provide direct services (https://www.samhsa.gov).

GLSMA grants require an evaluation plan, but the purpose of these grants is to fund programs and non-clinical services, not research. In terms of evaluating the funding program, the variety in program structure and data collection makes research challenging (Godoy Garraza et al., 2018). Nonetheless, some evaluations have provided insights into the context-specific needs of suicide prevention programs and site readiness for programs. Across sites, students who are suicidal often drop out of treatment, and there is a need for additional research[4] on how to engage at-risk students for treatment and lower barriers to receiving services (Godoy Garraza et al., 2018).

Over the past 15 years, GLSMA has focused most of its funding on supporting interventions to increase help-seeking by students or increase the community's ability to successfully identify and refer students in need. These themes are consistent with the original suicide prevention focus of the bill. However, because these interventions are designed to increase the number of students seeking mental health services (and thus preventing suicide), it is possible that some of the increase in demand for services being observed nationally is a result of interventions such as this. Future funding decisions will need to proactively align intervention efforts with growing clinical capacity to receive students who are identified and referred for help.

MENTAL HEALTH AND SUBSTANCE USE SERVICES AND STAFF

The range of clinical services that college and university centers provide varies substantially. For example, evidence-based treatments such as psychotherapy may not be available everywhere (IOM, 2015). According to ACCA, the majority of support takes the form of one-on-one therapy sessions, group counseling, testing and assessment, and emergency services (College Counseling Knowledge-Base: Comprehensive Database of College Counseling Research Publications in the College Counseling, Counseling Psychology, College Health, College Student Development and Professional Counseling Literatures 1998-2017) (see Chapter 3 for more information on general, non-clinical programs and services). Students who can benefit from short-term therapy might meet regularly with a therapist at the campus counseling center. For those students in need of long-term therapy or who have mental health issues beyond the scope of what the campus counseling staff can offer, a center can make referrals to local providers; however, issues related to off-campus providers can limit the degree to which students can access services (Brown, 2020). (Please see below for a section on Referrals to External and Community Providers and Chapter 5 for more information on referrals.)

The Association of University and College Counseling Center Directors' 2019 survey of 562 university and college counseling center directors found

---

[4] Chapter 6 lays out a proposed research agenda.

that "37.2 percent of counseling centers used a version of stepped care, offering a campus-wide menu of service options ranging from no care at all to weekly therapy at the counseling center. Depending on the center, options may include appropriate forms of self-help, wellness coaching, support groups, mindfulness classes, appropriate apps and online resources, etc." (LeViness et al., 2019). In addition, 46.6 percent of counseling center directors reported that psychiatric services are offered on their campus, and 57 percent of directors whose centers have psychiatric services reported that they need more hours of psychiatric services than they currently have to meet student needs (LeViness et al., 2019).

While the overall model may be similar, the range of services, hours and locations, and the number and expertise of staff available at a given institution can vary considerably. The staffing model at an institution's counseling center may include but is not limited to psychiatrists, counselors, other therapists, case workers, campus outreach coordinators, training directors, liaisons to community providers, group programming coordinators, student advisors, and graduate students in psychology, psychiatry, and social work. Staffing for centers continues to grow; the AUCCCD survey found that 43.9 percent of centers added staff positions between 2018 and 2019, while only 5.1 percent lost staff positions during the same time period.

Community colleges do not necessarily follow the same trends and may face a different set of expectations, as 96 percent of counselors in community colleges have other duties such as academic advising, career counseling, and other administrative duties (IACS, 2019). State licensing bodies for psychology, counseling, and social work may vary as well.

Community colleges may not have the same ability to dedicate funding to support mental health services and staff as more well-funded institutions, as they are less likely to have financial support from states and lack the security of the endowment funds that have safeguarded wealthy institutions. Community colleges tend to serve students from lower socio-economic backgrounds and have fewer options for recourse in terms of raising funds. In particular, these colleges may have dual-role counselors tasked with providing academic advising and general counseling to the student (Eisenberg et al., 2016). In a 2017 survey of community colleges in 30 states concerning dual-role staff, 51 percent of these staff provide academic advising (in addition to mental health counseling), and 73 percent provide mental health counseling in the same office where other student services are provided (Edwards and Lenhart, 2017). Some 66 percent of counseling center directors reported providing psychiatric services, and 56 percent of these directors report needing more hours of psychiatric services to meet the student need (IACS, 2019; LeViness et al., 2019)

Historically Black Colleges and Universities (HBCUs) and Tribal Colleges and Universities (TCUs) face similar challenges in terms of receiving less financial support from states. HBCUs and TCUs, along with community colleges, provide education to a broader group of students, have lower tuition and fees, provide more flexibility and accommodations for working students, and services that provide an environment inclusive to Black and Indigenous students.

Similarly, several HBCUs and TCUs and other colleges and universities have a limited ability to provide psychiatric services to students. Some of the impediments are financial, such as lack of funding for a full-time position and only being able to offer limited hours and a part-time position, while others might be related to the more widespread paucity of psychiatrists in the community. In terms of access, the result is that students who need psychiatric evaluations, treatment, and oversight to manage medical approaches often do not have access on campus and given the general shortage of psychiatrists in the nation, may not have access to a community provider either (Pedrelli et al., 2015). Of the universities that can afford to have an on-campus psychiatrist, many have only one—and time constraints often limit their role to medication evaluation and management and crisis evaluation (Iarovici, 2014). Of the centers that offer psychiatric services, 56.3 percent reported that there is more demand than their current level of services can address. For students who require medications as a part of their treatment, challenges may arise identifying a psychiatrist on campus or in the community. Just as in the community, colleges and universities rely increasingly on primary care providers to step in and provide pharmacological treatments to students with mental health issues.

One limiting factor for staffing of campus counseling centers is compensation. Compensation in higher education positions tends to be lower than in other sectors, which often means that qualified applicants have the option of leaving for higher-paying positions elsewhere (LeViness et al., 2019). Other factors making it difficult to staff centers include burnout resulting from high caseloads and lack of flexibility in determining schedules as compared with private practice settings (Kafka, 2019).

Referrals to External and Community Providers

Depending on the scope of care and available services at a college or university mental health center, campuses may provide students with off-campus referrals. Centers may offer students information about community clinics, local hospitals, or formal or informal referral channels to private providers. However, the shift from a college counseling center to an external provider can present challenges for exchange of records, finding a provider, scheduling, insurance coverage and cost, transportation, and student comfort (King Lyn, 2015). In terms of student comfort, individuals with some historically excluded identities may feel comfortable seeking services on a campus if they feel a sense of belonging; however, depending on the surrounding region, some students may not be as willing to leave campus. Even for community colleges students who may not have the same connection to a physical campus, these institutions are more likely to serve students who have had less access to mental health resources and may seek support from a place they are already know and trust. This may include students who are BIPOC in predominantly white areas or SGM students in states that have been hostile to people with their identities. The awareness that some communities may not feel welcoming or inclusive can help staff at some centers understand why students may not wish to seek off-campus services and work with students to update their centers' resources and guidance accordingly.

There is also great variability in the availability of appropriate service providers in the communities surrounding institutions of higher education (King Lyn, 2015). To ease the process referring students, college and university mental health staff may build connections to local providers, refer students to practices where there are existing connections, and provide students with information about two-way communication that can occur between the campus center and external provider with a release of information. Other ways to support the process may include information about how to look for providers based on insurance; how to understand co-pays, costs, and providers with sliding scales; providers that offer extended hours, speak other languages, or have specialties related to specific identities or health issues; and ways to address frequently asked questions or misconceptions related to off-site care. Some colleges and universities have begun hiring case workers and other staff positions to help students navigate and manage off-campus services.

Additional challenges with off-campus services relate to the availability of psychological, therapeutic, and psychiatric services in the local community and region. Rural communities across the United States have seen a decline in general health care providers and have struggled to have medical providers of all specialties serve in more remote areas. Some urban areas have been historically limited in their access to health care as a result of bias in public funding; unwillingness of medical providers to work in neighborhoods that predominantly serve individuals who are BIPOC; and discriminatory urban planning. For students at campuses in communities with limited mental health resources, off-campus services may require long waiting periods and other barriers related to overwhelmed providers. It is also worth noting that not all health care services are equal, and students may determine that the available services do not merit the potential costs of seeking treatment. See Chapter 5 for recommendations for ways to address these issues.

Substance Use Treatment, Substance Use Recovery Programs, and Programs for Students in Recovery

The National Institute on Alcohol Abuse and Alcoholism published the College Alcohol Intervention Matrix (CollegeAIM) in 2015 to help college personnel create comprehensive, campus-specific alcohol intervention strategies. CollegeAIM provides a range of individual- and environmental-level policy options aimed at reducing underage and excessive drinking among college students. These policies are ranked in CollegeAIM according to effectiveness, evidence-base, and cost; each policy is accompanied by information on barriers to effectiveness, the staffing required for policy enactment and implementation, and other factors. The authors of CollegeAIM emphasize that a mix of strategies is the best method to maximize positive effects and reduce excessive drinking and related problems among college students. Examples of the types of interventions included in the CollegeAIM matrix are:

- Enforcement of the age-21 drinking age
- Establishment of minimum unit pricing of alcoholic beverages and increasing the alcohol tax
- Prohibiting alcohol use and sales at campus sporting events and restricting alcohol sponsorship and advertising
- Retaining a ban on Sunday sales (where applicable) and limiting the number and density of alcohol establishments
- Conducting campus-wide social norms campaigns
- Personalized normative feedback programs that provide all students with information about their alcohol use in comparison with actual use by their peers

These strategies, practices, and policies are consistent with the Surgeon General's Call to Action and 2016 Report on Alcohol, Drugs, and Health.

Another resource, *The Guide to Best Practices,* published by the Maryland Collaborative to Reduce Underage Drinking and Related Problems (MCRCDRP, 2013), similarly summarizes individual- and environmental-level strategies available to college campuses. At the individual level, the authors advise that campuses should develop a roadmap outlining how they screen for and identify students in need of services, and refer them to necessary treatment. This roadmap should state how institutions will provide training to key individuals on campus, use valid and reliable screening instruments, track student screening and identification, and engage parents in all stages of the student's college career. At the environmental level, the guide asserts that campuses should build coalitions with the wider community, be proactive in enforcing existing alcohol laws, reduce the density of alcohol outlets near campus, address alcohol pricing and other promotional practices, and incorporate community-enhancing practices into landlord lease agreements.

Since the 1970s, colleges and universities have introduced collegiate recovery programs (CRPs) to support students with substance use disorders (Hazelden Betty Ford Foundation, 2020). While all institutions of higher education are required to conduct prevention and education efforts to reduce the presence of illegal and dangerous alcohol consumption for students, "most are lacking in specific programming to support those students who are in recovery" (The Ohio State University, 2020). CRPs can provide integrated services for students in recovery with a combination of academic and health-oriented approaches. While services vary across providers, common features may include "substance-free housing and social events, dedicated space, on-campus twelve-step support meetings, full-time dedicated staff and professional counseling by addiction treatment specialists" (Hazelden Betty Ford Foundation, 2020). Some colleges and universities may require students to sign contracts to participate in these programs that include minimum standards for academic performance, sobriety, and participation in programs to remain eligible, while others are barrier-free and welcome all of those in recovery or in search of recovery (Hazelden Betty Ford Foundation, 2020).

CRPs are intended to support students who arrive on campus already in recovery as well as students who develop substance use disorders during their enrollment. Research estimates that approximately 250,000 students in higher education have received treatment for substance use in their lifetime (Hazelden Betty Ford Foundation, 2020). At present, there are approximately 100 schools who have joined the Association of Recovery in Higher Education with commitments to CRPs through the Transforming Youth Recovery effort (The Ohio State University, 2020). However, the increase in programs does not necessarily mean that treatment for all substance use issues has grown evenly: "Although many initiatives target active substance abuse problems on campus, particularly binge drinking, few services are available that specifically aid students in recovery from alcohol or drug addiction" (Perron et al., 2011).

CRPs and other programs may likely work best with colleges and universities that have a large on-campus population. Community colleges, some graduate programs, and virtual universities may face different challenges, and there is little research on substance use prevention and treatment specific to these populations. For community colleges, there are studies that correlate the increased number of students who have experienced an adverse childhood experience (see Chapter 3 for more on Student Survivors of Trauma) with both community college enrollment and substance use disorders (Cadigan and Lee, 2019).

Challenges and Opportunities in Utilizing Telehealth to Support Mental Health Services

Telehealth refers to a variety of methods of synchronous or asynchronous communication with a mental health professional via video conferencing, email, text, online chat tools, or the phone (Higher Education Mental Health Alliance, 2014). Telehealth services, which is a form of distance therapy offered by a mental health provider directly via online mechanisms, should not be confused with other online programs and virtual applications that support students with the goal of general wellbeing or stress management (see Chapter 3). The most popular services were mental health screening online (27.5 percent) and telephone counseling (7.6 percent) (LeViness et al., 2019). While existing research focuses on synchronous delivery through video-conference platforms, which best simulate a face-to-face session, there is less information on new models of delivery such as text support or the use of third-party psychoeducational and self-help tools. (Higher Education Mental Health Alliance, 2014).

The COVID-19 pandemic has rapidly transformed both the treatment of mental health problems as well as the promotion of mental health, through the use of telehealth services. Prior to the pandemic, the American Psychiatric Association reported that most of its member clinicians did not use telehealth; however, as of June 2020, 85 percent said that they were serving more than three-quarters of their patients through telehealth (American Psychological Association, 2020). Telehealth services have also permitted students from many campuses to engage in group psychotherapy during COVID-19, mitigating mental health consequences of forced relocation, social distancing, and isolation. Similarly, according to a 2019 survey report from the Association of University and College Counseling Center Directors, greater than 50 percent of college counseling center directors said their center used no form of telehealth, and only 3.4 percent of the directors surveyed said they offered counseling via videoconferencing (LeViness et al., 2019). With COVID-19, the rapid expansion of these services has been seen on and off campus. With this expansion comes the need to understand the challenges and opportunities associated with these services; telehealth offers the safest opportunity in terms of COVID-19 risks for seeking health care in this moment and during the foreseeable future and will likely continue to expand and transform health care delivery. As a recent report notes, given that telehealth will likely continue to be a health service delivery mechanism beyond the pandemic, "it will be important for universities to identify and make available the best telehealth resources and incorporate them into [the] college or university's health strategy" (Steve Fund, 2020). Under normal circumstances, telehealth services can be a method to support students who attend a college or university virtually, who are off-campus for a semester abroad or while conducting research, or for those who have life circumstances (e.g., conflicting schedules, transportation issues, and disability) that preclude them from visiting in-person services (Higher Education Mental Health Alliance, 2019). However, while this mode of delivery may increase access for some students, other groups of services may not provide the same benefits as in-person sessions, posing significant issues of equity. For example, students who have challenges accessing the internet or lack adequate devices may not be able to benefit from these services. Other students may lack a private space for accessing these services, either on or off campus. Access to telehealth services is a significant challenge. Opportunities to increase access may include providing students with a private space and access to high speed internet to support telehealth sessions. There may also be students who choose one delivery method over another because of personal preference alone. Finally, it is important to note that many tele-mental-health companies employ a wide variety of "rule-outs" when determining who is appropriate for their services (e.g., drug abuse, suicidality, serious mental illness) that will limit access for many students.

In the wake of COVID-19, access to distance and tele-services has allowed many students to remain in touch with their on-campus counselors. This is a noteworthy shift, as one of the major issues that had limited students from getting teletherapy with an existing provider was the limitation of providing services across state or international boundaries, due to restrictions imposed by licensing boards and legislation. After the pandemic began, many states began to grant waivers to health care providers to provide tele-services. Penn State University and the University of Texas at Austin compiled and updated an omnibus guide on the changing rules/laws in each state related to providing mental health services via telehealth/telemedicine across state lines (CHMC, 2020).[5] The future of the laws and regulations remains uncertain at the time of publication of this report. For more information about research questions related to telehealth, see Chapter 6.

While there is evidence that the provision of mental health services via telehealth has expanded greatly during the pandemic, the relative effectiveness of these services has not yet been well documented. Several studies of the application of telehealth services on campus prior to the pandemic have indicated that this may be an effective mechanism for reaching more students. Nobleza et al. (2018), for example, examined the telehealth experience of students in a college counseling center prior to the pandemic. Participants were health professional students who utilized at least one telehealth visit between November 2015 and April 2017 and were surveyed to assess the impact of telehealth on access, experience, effectiveness, and impact on therapeutic alliance. The majority of the 53.7 percent of students who responded indicated that telehealth was convenient (94.4 percent), time-saving (94.4 percent), and helped them to feel better (83.3 percent). The authors noted that "eighty-one percent reported telehealth as being as good, nearly as good, or no different than meeting in person... telehealth is a viable option for college counseling centers and is experienced as convenient, time-saving, and effective with little negative impact on therapeutic alliance." (King et al., 2019).

Similarly, King et al. (2019) studied the effectiveness of a well-validated tool, termed the brief alcohol screening and intervention for college students (BASICS) when conducted face-to-face or through a videoconferencing system. The authors found that that the intervention "significantly reduced alcohol consumption and related problems regardless of condition." King et al. (2019) also noted that the study suggested that "telehealth services should be further implemented and the BASICS intervention can be effectively delivered via telehealth for college students."

---

[5] The second version expanded the range of health care professionals, and it now includes marriage and family therapists, physicians, professional counselors, psychologists, and social workers, as well as advanced practice nurses, physician assistants, and physical therapists.

Despite initial positive evidence that telehealth may increase access to both mental health treatment and wellness services, further study with the advent of COVID-19 and the acceleration of these services is needed. In addition to understanding challenges associated with accessing services, research should examine the effectiveness of telehealth compared to standard in-person approaches, especially for specific populations.

5

Moving Forward

As emphasized throughout this report, there is an urgent need to attend to student mental health and substance use because (1) they are critical factors in determining student success (Eisenberg, Golberstein, and Gollust, 2009; Shankar and Park, 2016; Topham and Moller, 2011), (2) students at all types of institutions of higher education and in all fields of study are reporting increasing numbers of problems with mental health and substance use (Lattie, Lipson, Eisenberg, 2019), and (3) colleges are consistently reporting that the demand for mental health services exceeds the supply. The increased prevalence of mental health and substance use problems has many academic leaders and policymakers describing the situation in near-crisis terms and looking for solutions.

This chapter aims to provide those leaders, as well as agencies that fund efforts to improve student mental health, with evidence-based approaches for addressing the major issues confronting institutions as they try to meet the growing demand for mental health and substance use services among their students, building on the already proven effectiveness of campus counseling centers (McAleavey et al., 2017). The challenge for the committee in offering these approaches is that there can be no one-size-fits-all solutions given the diversity of institutions, their institutional and financial capacities, and their specific student populations. For example, a community college with a predominantly commuter student body is likely to encounter a very different constellation of issues and have different resources available to deal with them than a four-year university. Within other groups, such as large public land-grant institutions, HBCUs and TCUs, and liberal arts colleges, each institution will need to find strategies to support its unique populations without regressing to the modal demographic group and identities. There are also enormous differences among the students who attend these colleges and universities with respect to financial resources, access to health care, whether they have health insurance, and, if they do, the quality of those health plans. Research has also documented differences in the prevalence of symptoms and use of services across race and ethnicity, socioeconomic background, gender identity, and academic discipline (Eisenberg, Hunt, and Speer, 2013; Lipson et al., 2016). When appropriate, this chapter points out interventions designed for specific types of institutions or student populations as well.

In the committee's judgment, based on its information gathering activities, there are multiple proven approaches for intervening around mental health and substance use issues and promoting student wellbeing in ways that will positively affect student success. For that reason, the committee is not advocating a single "ideal" that all institutions of higher education should adopt or strive for. Rather, the committee includes in this chapter a discussion of the major issues confronting institutions of higher education as they strive to better meet students' needs and ways those problems or barriers to progress might be addressed.

INSTITUTIONAL CULTURE AND POLICIES

Institutions of higher education must establish and/or maintain a culture that accepts and supports, to the extent possible, students experiencing problems with mental health and substance use and fosters a sense of wellbeing for all students. For some institutions, this will require a significant culture shift. The culture starts with the institution's leadership—the president and board of trustees. Without institutional support and leadership, progress in providing needed supports may allow too many students with problems to fall through the cracks. The Okanagan Charter is one useful guide that can help colleges and universities embed health into all aspects of campus culture and climate, as well as promote collaborative action to create a health-promoting environment (Okanagan Charter, 2015).[1]

Changing Institutional Culture

Developing a Campus Culture Focused on Wellbeing

The committee acknowledges how difficult it is to change any organizational culture and climate, and those within institutions of higher education are no different. Nonetheless, the committee recognizes that accomplishing difficult tasks is a hallmark of the U.S. higher education enterprise (see Box 5-1). One framework for culture change, known as collective impact, requires that everyone on campus shares a common agenda, is provided with a coordinating structure, engages in mutually reinforcing activities, participates in continuous communication, and

---

[1] Additional information is available at https://collegehealthqi.nyu.edu/20x30/frameworks/okanagan-charter (accessed April 29, 2020).

BOX 5-1
Defining Organizational Climate and Culture

While organizational climate is focused on the shared perceptions within an organization, organizational culture is defined as "the collectively held beliefs, assumptions, and values held by organizational members" (Stamarski and Hing, 2015, p. 7; see also Trice and Beyer, 1993, Settles et al., 2006, and Schein, 2010). Ideally, the climate reflects and supports the culture of the organization, and ideally, the culture guides and sets the tone for the climate that members of an organization experience. The key is that climate and culture must be addressed together, because efforts to build a good climate will flounder if they conflict with the beliefs, assumptions, and values of an organization; conversely, only having the "right" culture will not result in the desired result if the processes and procedures are not organized around the collective and shared goals and beliefs (Schneider, Ehrhart, and Macey, 2013).

To address culture change in an organization, it is crucial to recognize that organizational cultures are not neutral. Rather, they reflect the norms and values of those who are and have been in leadership roles in the organizations, and these norms influence the formal and informal structures, organizational strategy, human resource systems, and organizational climates (Gelfand, Erez, and Aycan, 2007). As a result, organizational culture change cannot be addressed in isolation. Further, organizational leadership, and the signals that leaders send about civility, respect, and tolerance for sexual harassment, are powerful cues that individuals in the organization take seriously—and they adapt their own behaviors (if not their attitudes) accordingly.

Source: NASEM, 2018b.

---

agrees on shared measurement systems to evaluate and boost progress (Christens and Inzeo, 2015; Poleman, Jenkes-Jay, and Bryne, 2019; Slusser et al., 2018). The committee believes that general approach applies here.

The committee also believes that the unequal impacts of the COVID-19 pandemic and the call to action in response to the killing of Black men and women by police reflect the long-standing disparities that BIPOC and those of low socioeconomic status experience daily in American society. The protests and public outcry in response to these events have created an environment in which the public may be more willing to engage in further steps toward dismantling racism and systemic oppression. It is in the spirit of this moment that the committee believes that academic leaders have an important role to play in bringing together the different communities on campus to address those aspects of institutional culture that do not support the mental health and wellbeing of all students, particularly students who are BIPOC or who come from other underrepresented groups.

RECOMMENDATION 5-1

Institutional leaders, starting with the president and board of trustees or regents, should articulate the importance of creating a culture of wellbeing on their campus, one that recognizes the range of individual behaviors and community norms that affect wellbeing, acknowledges the magnitude of mental health and substance use issues on campus, addresses the stigma associated with mental illness and substance use disorders, and provides a range of resources to support students with different levels of need.

The stakeholders required to create and/or maintain this kind of culture must go beyond the administrators, counseling center staff, and offices within student affairs. It requires the entire faculty,[2] staff, and student body working together to recognize the importance of the following (Byrd and McKinney, 2012; Chen, Romero, and Karver, 2016):

- validating, respecting, and supporting individuals in all their identities,
- attending to the demand for mental health and substance use services that now exists and is likely to grow,
- proactively addressing student mental health and substance use,
- creating and/or sustaining a campus culture and environment that minimizes stress and promotes the emotional wellness of everyone on campus,
- discussing, acknowledging, and acting to correct existing systems that harm individuals and pose risks to their wellbeing

Creating and Sustaining Cross-Campus Coordination, Collaboration, and Leadership That Support a Culture of Wellbeing

One approach that institutions have used to address other cross-campus concerns such as diversity, equity, and inclusion efforts; mentoring and teaching; and security concerns on campus has been to establish a campus-wide action commission with representatives from faculty, students, staff, and administrative units. These action commissions have an effective leadership structure (it may be a single leader or a small group, depending on the needs of the institution) and a clear charge to build or maintain a culture that supports student wellbeing. Thus, a standing, campus-wide commission might be one such mechanism for creating a campus culture that supports students' mental health and wellbeing. This approach can be a strong first step toward ensuring there is cross-unit

---

[2] Faculty here include tenure- and non-tenure track faculty, as well as adjunct faculty, part-time faculty, lecturers, and other instructors, with admission that many of these positions do not receive the same kind of training, support, and benefits as full-time, tenure-track faculty. Additionally, community colleges and other colleges and universities that have a higher percentage of adjunct faculty, part-time faculty, lecturers, or other instructors may not have received the same kind of professional development and support as their full-time, tenure-track peers.

communication and collective buy-in to promote culture change and establish a compact of shared responsibility.

RECOMMENDATION 5-2
Leadership from all segments of the campus community is needed to promote a culture of wellbeing.
- Institutions of higher education should establish and/or maintain a team or teams that involves all sectors of the institution's community that coordinates, reviews, and addresses mental health, substance use, and wellbeing concerns.
- Any approach should have shared responsibility for addressing issues that negatively affect student wellbeing, a clear leadership structure and mandate, appropriate access to financial resources, and a charge to develop and implement an action plan to promote and support student wellbeing.

One troublesome aspect of societal culture in the United States, which is also present at our institutions, is the pernicious stigma surrounding mental illness and substance use. Addressing stigma is a critical component in promoting mental health and wellbeing among all students. For an individual, the stigma related to mental illness and substance use issues has a number of possible influences, including their family's views and history; interpretations and lessons from cultural, religious, and spiritual connections; social norms; and their peer group's beliefs and actions (NASEM, 2016). General efforts to reduce stigma around mental health and substance use programs aimed at all students through awareness campaigns and wellbeing efforts are one way to combat the impact of stigma. See Box 5-2 for an example of an evidence-based mental health treatment program.

As colleges and universities seek to end the stigma tied to mental illness and substance use, institutions of higher education should review how their own systems may enhance stigma, create barriers, or otherwise fail to serve students from groups that have not been well-served by mental health services in the past. Many colleges and universities, as well the broader U.S. health care system, have long had both direct or implicit biases against BIPOC, women, SGM individuals, and people with many other identities. Given these historic barriers and biases (DeLisa and Lindenthal, 2012; Harrison-Bernard et al., 2020; Nivet, 2015; Ong et al., 2011), campuses must ensure that their current services welcome, respect, and provide inclusive services to all students. This includes providing services for students who return to campus as older adults, as well as those with dependents and those who have served in the military. As noted later in this chapter, the Equity in Mental Health Framework, developed by the Jed Foundation, the Steve Fund, and McLean Hospital's College Mental Health Program, is an accessible resource for schools seeking to promote mental health and wellbeing among students of color and other underrepresented student populations (Steve Fund and Jed Foundation, 2017). This framework provides academic institutions with a set

---

BOX 5-2
McLean Hospital College Mental Health Program

Each year, the McLean Hospital College Mental Health Program (CMHP) supports more than 200 different colleges and universities in addressing a range of issues and psychiatric illnesses, including executive functioning, anxiety, depression, obsessive-compulsive disorder, eating concerns, and substance use. The program model focuses on working closely with college student-patients, their families, and their institutions of higher education,

For students receiving treatment throughout McLean Hospital, CMHP works with students and their institutions of higher education, providing students a variety of supports, including symptom education groups, consultation to treatment teams, and individual meetings with students planning to return to college or preparing to take a medical leave of absence. The program offers academic consultation, transition support, and outpatient services to students who are struggling to co-manage their mental health and academic lives.

Services are open to students currently enrolled in college, on a leave of absence from school, or seeking support in their transition to college for the first time. The program offers support for students, including tools to support students experiencing mental health conditions and recommendations related to on- and off-campus resources to support and enhance student well-being.

For more information, see https://www.mcleanhospital.org/treatment/cmhp.
Source: Steve Fund and Jed Foundation, 2017.

---

of 10 actionable recommendation, free resources, and supporting toolkits, as well as key implementation strategies to help strengthen their activities and programs to address the mental health disparities facing students of color and other underrepresented student populations, such as sexual and gender minorities (see Box 5-3 for specific framework case studies).

In developing the framework, the Steve Fund, Jed Foundation, and McLean Hospital's College Mental Health Program carried out a nationwide survey of campus programs intended to support mental health and wellbeing among students of color in an effort to identify promising practices. The framework organizes these promising practices in a five-tiered structure based on the extent to which a program: (1) had a specific focus on mental health and emotional wellbeing; (2) had a specific focus on college, graduate, or professional students of color; and (3) utilized evidence-based practices. The survey identified a single tier 1 program out of a total of 84 programs that included both an empirical evidence base and a specific focus on mental health in students of color (see Box 5-3 for a description of the tier 1 program and several tier 2 programs). The report writes: "Whereas the majority of programs had collected some type of data (typically, qualitative feedback or student satisfaction), the lack of systematic program

---

BOX 5-3
Case Studies from the Mental Health Equity Framework

CASE STUDY EXAMPLE: At Connecticut College, a facilitator-led program called Empowerment Through Mindfulness teaches mindfulness skills within a student group (SHE Sister Program) for women of color including faculty, staff, and students. After teaching core evidence-based mindfulness principles, the group completes guided exercises around cultural pride, resilience, affirmation, and related empowerment. The Mental Health Equity Framework considers this program a tier 1 program in that it includes an empirical evidence base and a specific focus on mental health in students of color. It is the only program in the framework categorized as tier 1.

CASE STUDY EXAMPLE: The University of Vermont hosts a retreat called "Racial Aikido"' co-hosted by the Center for Cultural Pluralism and the ALANA Student Center. Topics of focus include recognizing race and racism in the United States, exploring racial/ethnic identities, responding to acts of racism, debunking stereotypes to maintain positive self-image, and healing from the impacts of racism. The Mental Health Equity Framework considers this program a tier 2 program because it has a focus on promoting emotional health and wellbeing in students of color and is supported by program evaluation or qualitative data.

CASE STUDY EXAMPLE: At the University of Florida, multicultural counseling staff and psychology department researchers are currently working together to develop a brief assessment battery for students engaged in one of its most highly attended 25 equityinmentalhealth.org programs (its Invincible Black Women group) over the past 10 years. These data will be used to better understand and disseminate outcomes of the program. The research team also plans to include other campus-level outcomes and to disseminate program materials so that other colleges and universities can readily implement similar programs. This program is also ranked as a tier 2 program by the Mental Health Equity Framework.

---

development efforts left the questions of efficacy and effectiveness unanswered in the vast majority of these tailored interventions."

There is a clear need for additional research on strategies and practices that can support the mental health and well-being of students of color. Nevertheless, the committee endorses the use of the Mental Health Equity Framework as a foundation for practice and encourages each individual campus to set additional priorities, strategies, and actions to ensure an equitable and inclusive culture.

CHANGING INSTITUTIONAL POLICIES

Policies for Medical Leave and Re-enrollment

Institutional medical leave and reenrollment policies, when they exist, can serve as barriers for students whose mental health or substance use problems are severe enough that they lead the student to withdraw from school at least temporarily. Many institutions limit how long a student's leave of absence can last before they must reapply for readmission. In addition, withdrawal from school can affect financial aid. However, the Americans with Disabilities Act (ADA) mandates that students with disabilities, including those related to mental health and substance use, have the right to reasonable accommodations for their disability. Such accommodations include extra time on exams or assignments, the ability to withdraw from specific classes, and leaves of absence that allow for reenrollment (Martin, 2017). The COVID-19 pandemic has also highlighted the ability for higher education to adopt virtual tools and other teaching modalities that may continue to accommodate students with disabilities.

Since 2011, the Department of Education's Office of Civil Rights, which is responsible for enforcing ADA provisions, has allowed institutions of higher education to require an involuntary medical leave for students with a mental health issue. The proviso indicates that students must be allowed to reenroll in school upon providing certification from a medical professional that they are fit to return to the school community (see Box 5-4). Students who take a voluntary medical leave for a mental health issue should also be allowed to reenroll in school under the same proviso. In the event that a student returns to campus and has ongoing mental health issues, learning disabilities, or other challenges covered by the ADA, the campus is required to provide academic accommodations and make reasonable modifications of policies to remove barriers for the student (Baselon et al., 2008).

An important step toward creating an integrated approach to supporting students would be to establish a closer collaboration between academic affairs and student affairs. While every campus has a different arrangement of staff and division of responsibilities, campuses that build an intentional bridge between academic and student affairs increase the chances for students with mental health concerns or substance use to succeed (Nesheim et al., 2007).

RECOMMENDATION 5-3
Institutions should ensure that their leave of absence and reenrollment policies and practices will accommodate the needs of students experiencing mental health and substance use problems and the time needed for effective treatment and recovery.

- Institutions should implement methods to reduce and/or alleviate the financial burden on students related to medical leave and other issues related to course completion.
- Academic affairs and student affairs units should develop collaborations to share information appropriately, while also respecting a student's right to private/confidential treatment, in order to support students at the intersection of mental health and academic concerns.

BOX 5-4
Students Returning from Medical Leave

Students who experience significant life events, illness, or substance issues may choose to leave campus to receive specialized treatment, to tend to family or other dependents, or to dedicate time to health and healing. Students who take a medical leave of absence for any reason may wish to consider the following questions when developing a plan to return to campus. The following guidance may also be helpful for incoming students to review before arriving on campus. The following suggestions have been adapted from the National Association of State Mental Health Program Directors guide, *Back to School: Toolkits to Support the Full Inclusion of Students with Early Psychosis in Higher Education*:

- Continuation of care: For students who have received medical treatment and health services at a separate location, devising a plan for continued support through remote support or planned appointments during breaks to ensure continuity is important.
- Referrals to local services: Research on services available through the campus health service or through local, private providers can help inform a transition plan. Working to establish connections prior to arrival, including releases of information with previous providers if necessary, can ease the return. Even for students who have recovered, a transition plan may include a list of available health care services and providers in the event of an emergency.
- Understanding previous events: For students who have experienced events precipitated by certain circumstances or factors, a plan may include ways to anticipate issues and methods to address them as needed.
- Communication with family or off-campus support networks: For individuals who have emergency contacts away from campus, a plan may include frequency of communication with updates and check-ins regarding health. Depending on the health issue, emergency contacts may wish to establish a protocol if they have not heard from the student. Students may also explore and consider signing a waiver to release health information to emergency contacts in the event arises.
- Students services and disability accommodations: For students who would benefit from accommodations, the Americans with Disabilities Act requires that students self-identify and provide documentation to receive formal accommodations. In the event a student has not registered a formal documentation, accommodations cannot be provided in case symptoms arise unexpectedly (Jones et al., 2016b).

PRIORITIZING MENTAL HEALTH AMID
FINANCIAL CONSTRAINTS

As the committee noted in Chapter 1, and emphasized again here, the U.S. postsecondary educational system is one of the few systems in the nation, other than the military, whose stakeholders expect to provide low-cost or free treatment for those within its community with mental health and substance use problems. When the costs of providing that care rise, colleges and universities have few options to keep pace. Raising tuition or reallocating resources from other campus priorities are two such options, but both have proven unpopular with stakeholders. Academic institutions are therefore caught between the need to expend more resources on student wellbeing while not increasing the overall cost of education.

Economic pressures increased operating costs, and greater market competition are an ever-increasing set of challenges for U.S. institutions of higher education. A 2014 survey of college and university board chairs and presidents, for example, found that about 60 percent believe the financial stability of higher education is moving in the wrong direction (Selingo, 2015). This situation has been made worse by the COVID-19 pandemic, which forced colleges and universities to effectively close their campuses for educational and research purposes and move to online instruction in the spring of 2020. In addition, the report notes that the cost of student services and student facilities, such as campus counseling centers, represent a major concern to university presidents.

Tuition revenues have plateaued in recent years, with Moody's Investor Services reporting that flat enrollment, rising tuition discount rates, and an emphasis on affordability contributed to limited growth in net tuition revenues (McCabe and Fitzgerald, 2019).[3] For public universities and community colleges, declines in federal, state, and local support are further stressing budgets. Forbes, in its sixth report on the financial health of private, not-for-profit colleges, reported that "the overall financial wellbeing of colleges has deteriorated and many are in danger of closing or merging" (Schifrin and Coudriet, 2019). Prior to the start of the pandemic, the largest community college system in Pennsylvania eliminated its counseling service, despite the acknowledgement of need, due to loss of funding related to declines in student tuition and eliminating licensed counselors with the intent to bring on student advisors with a greater focus on career planning (Anderson, 2019). Moreover, the COVID-19 pandemic is causing further financial stresses for many of the nation's colleges and universities (Associated Press, 2020; Capatides, 2020; Pannett, 2020). In spite of these economic pressures, the committee believes that mental health, substance use, and wellbeing issues are sufficiently important that increased funding will have to be devoted to them.

---

[3] Net tuition revenue is a key financial indicator since it serves as the foundation for most college and university budgets. Financial pressure mounts on an institution if its net tuition revenue does not rise as quickly as expenses or inflation.

Prioritizing Funding and Services for Mental Health on Campus

RECOMMENDATION 5-4

Institutions of higher education and the government agencies that support them should increase the priority given to funding for campus and community mental health and substance use services.

- National, state, and local funders of higher education should incentivize colleges and universities to effectively provide support for students' mental health and substance use problems.
- In their budgets, hiring, programming, expectations for serving students, and assessment/evaluation activities, institutions should make mental health a higher priority on campus. They should also work more directly with state and local governments, where relevant, to help bring this about.
- To ensure that mental health and emotional wellness services are prioritized, institutions should consider reallocating existing institutional funds to support counseling centers, support the increased use of online mental health services (when appropriate), and support data collection on the need for and use of mental health services by students.
- Institutions should actively collaborate with local health care services and facilities and community providers, for example, by considering hiring staff to help students navigate and manage off-campus services.

States should modify insurance laws or regulations, or provide administrative guidance, to enable institutions to use general funds and/or designated health fees for expenses that are not covered by students' personal insurance.

Making a Value Case for Addressing Student Mental Health Problems

The assumption that bolstering the capacity of the counseling and psychological services centers and creating other programs aimed at improving student mental health only adds to existing financial burdens is not necessarily true given that colleges and universities lose revenue when students drop out because of mental health or substance use problems. A 2018 survey by the Association for University and College Counseling Center Directors (AUCCCD) found that "counseling services have a positive impact on retention, as measured by student self-report," with 63.2 percent of counseling center clients reporting that counseling services helped them stay in school (LeViness et al., 2018). Other studies have also documented this relationship between counseling services and student retention, including Lee et al. 2009, who conducted interviews and collected data on counseling services for a total of 10,009 students from a large public university in the northeastern United States. The authors found that "counseling experience is significantly associated with student retention: students receiving counseling services were more likely to stay enrolled in school."

In fact, public health economists associated with the Healthy Minds Network, based on research on the effectiveness of mental health care and on the economic returns to education, have calculated that a counseling center treating 500 students a year will help an average of 30 students remain enrolled in college (assuming a rate of $20,000 per student-year)—thereby increasing tuition revenues by $1.2 million over two years[4] (Samuels, 2019). In addition, by completing their degrees, those 30 students' lifetime earnings would increase by an estimated $3 million.[5] In addition to the monetary benefits of reducing attrition, accreditation services consider graduation rates in their reviews. By comparison, the researchers found that the "cost of providing mental health care for 500 depressed students would be no more than $500,000 based on standard estimates for the cost of psychiatric medication or brief models of psychotherapy" (HMN, 2013). Healthy Minds Network has created a return on investment tool that institutions of higher education can use to explore the economic benefits of investing in student mental health, which is available at http://healthymindsnetwork.org/research/roi-calculator. The tool includes assumptions that can be customized for the institution, for example, school population size, departure/retention rate, prevalence of depression, and alternative assumptions about the program's effectiveness in reducing depression (HMN, 2013).

Addressing Insurance Billing—One Approach for Raising Funds to Increase Capacity and Meet Demand

One option for funding mental health services is for colleges and universities to seek reimbursement by health plans for services rendered. Many colleges and universities require their students to have health insurance, yet few bill insurance companies for services rendered and instead cover the entire cost for those services themselves. A survey conducted by AUCCCD found that only 4.4 percent, of responding institutions billed third parties for their services (LeViness et al., 2018). There are many reasons that counseling centers do not bill insurance, including:

- concerns about student confidentiality when students are on their parents' insurance plan
- the cost involved in setting up billing infrastructure and credentialing providers
- the fact that many counseling centers have robust training programs that would have difficulty billing insurance
- concern about adding another barrier (cost) to seeking mental health care, especially for students and families with high deductible plans

---

[4] This assumes 60 student-years of tuition at $20,000 a year.
[5] This assumes an additional $50,000 per college year of earnings.

- the difficulty in some areas for mental health providers to get on insurance panels, and
- billing expenses exceeding returns, impact on training programs, the low reimbursement rates and burdensome requirements for pre-authorization for care, submission of treatment plans, and concurrent care review that drive many providers in the community from insurance panels in the first place.

The time, expense, and human resources needed to create the infrastructure to bill insurance companies is usually well beyond the capabilities of smaller institutions and community colleges. Moreover, colleges and universities that do not mandate that students have insurance coverage that meets specific requirements will have uninsured students who cannot afford services that require payment; even those that have insurance (from another state or with a particular carrier) may be out of network or otherwise challenged in paying for services while at college.

In the context of these concerns, the fact remains that many families already pay insurance carriers for coverage of services that colleges and universities provide, and that colleges and universities largely do not have access to these funds. Meanwhile, some institutions that do not bill for services struggle to adequately fund mental health service provision, while other institutions provide exceptional levels of service without billing. While institutions that do bill for services have added a revenue stream, they must still deal with the problem of increasing capacity to treat all students in need of services.

RECOMMENDATION 5-5
Institutions of higher education should work with insurance companies and health plans and federal, state, and local regulators to remove barriers to seeking reimbursement for student mental health and substance use costs for covered students.

- Insurance companies should keep up with market rates for reimbursement to incentivize more providers to accept insurance carried by students, support providers from institutions of higher education in becoming paneled quickly, and communicate and improve the confidentiality measures in place to dependent subscribers between the ages of 18-26 to ensure that they can seek services using their parents' insurance and be afforded the confidentiality they are entitled to receive.
- States should modify insurance laws or regulations, or provide administrative guidance, to enable institutions to use general funds and/or designated health fees for expenses that are not covered by students' personal insurance for charges incurred at student health and counseling services. This is commonly referred to as a secondary payor provision in coordination of benefits.

There are solutions to each of these issues, but they require action by state legislators and insurance regulators, and in some cases the federal government, to ensure that services provided by higher education institutions can be covered. For example, states that do not require health insurance for students could amend insurance laws to allow different charges for people with and without health insurance in higher education. State insurance regulations or university fee plans could also be changed to include additional privacy protections for adult dependents on their parents' health plans and to require insurance companies to empanel providers at colleges and universities that are delivering health services to their students.

UNDERSTANDING THE STATE OF STUDENT MENTAL HEALTH AND WELLBEING ON EACH CAMPUS

While colleges and universities share a similar set of challenges in supporting student mental health, the issues, priority areas, and available resources on campus vary substantially across institutions. In addition, every campus would benefit from identifying the local and regional mental health and substance use prevalence trends, service providers, and additional resources to fully inform referral practices, programming, and policies (Othman et al., 2019). Assessing the mental health and substance use treatment needs of a given population—a student body in this case—has been a significant problem and is different and more difficult than evaluating general "wellness." Surveys of incoming students can provide some baseline information related to a broader sense of wellbeing; however, these data have limited use in identifying specific mental health issues.

RECOMMENDATION 5-6
Institutions of higher education should conduct a regular assessment (preferably at least every two years) that addresses student mental health, substance use, wellbeing, and campus climate. The data generated from these assessments should be compared to peer institution data (as available for disaggregation). Analysts should create a data collection system that allows for disaggregation by unit, program level, and student identities. This assessment should include the extent that students are aware of and know how to access available resources, both on campus and in the local community, to address students' mental health and substance use problems.

- At the end of the academic year, institutions should review the many data points collected about their clinical trends and utilization as a way to understand how resources on campus can be used most effectively. These data would include the percentage of students who received treatment at the institution, the percentage that went outside of the institution for treatment, and the percentage of students that report needing help but did not seek or receive it, and should be further analyzed across demographic and identity groups.

- Funding agencies and private organizations should provide grants to under-resourced institutions, notably community colleges, Historically Black Colleges and Universities, and Tribal Colleges and Universities, to collect, analyze, and share data with the goal of implementing findings.

In addition to general climate assessment, there are a number of screening tools and instruments that colleges and universities can consider for assessing student mental health as a means of connecting students to mental health services before a crisis emerges. For example, the Counseling Center Assessment of Psychological Symptoms (CCAPS) instruments, developed by the Center for Collegiate Mental Health (CCMH) at Penn State University, is a frequently used measure for assessing mental health functioning of students seeking treatment through counseling centers (Locke et al., 2010). In addition, CCMH offers CCAPS-Screen, "a mental health screening instrument that assesses the most common psychological problems experienced ... including a critical item related to the report of suicidal ideation within the last two weeks."[6] Another set of measures and associated data can be found through the Healthy Minds Network. HMS also provides a campus-wide measure of student mental health and substance abuse issues, as well as a national assessment of mental health and substance abuse treatment needs (Lipson et al., 2019b).[7] Assessments of mental health literacy and peer-to-peer counseling referrals may be useful in the community college setting (Kalkbrenner, Sink, and Smith, 2020).

The American College Health Association's National College Health Assessment, an annual survey of college student health that includes mental health and substance abuse (Cain, 2018), provides a national perspective on the mental health and substance use issues that students face. In addition, the World Health Organization's World Mental Health International College Student (WMH-ICS) Initiative provides estimates of the prevalence of mental disorders, the adverse consequences on the personal, social, and academic levels of these disorders, patterns of help-seeking for these disorders, and barriers to treatment based on a representative sample of colleges and universities across the globe (Auerbach et al., 2018).

Beyond the screening tools described above, there are new methods for assessing the percentage of students who have mental health and substance use issues. One approach, for example, uses computerized adaptive testing (CAT), based on machine learning techniques, to determine what question from a

---

[6] Additional information is available at https://ccmh.psu.edu/ccaps-screen (accessed September 29, 2020).

[7] As noted in Chapter 1, the committee has found that much of the information on the incidence of mental health and substance use problems among students come from self-reports and not actual diagnoses by mental health professionals. Numerous investigators have pointed out that self-report data can be strongly biased and may not accurately reflect the true incidence of those issues among students in higher education (Dang, King, and Inzlicht, 2020).

large number of possible questions to ask an individual based on the answer to the proceeding question rather than having every individual answer every question included in an assessment vehicle. Using this technique, researchers have developed the CAT-mental health (CAT-MH) suite of 10 CAT. (Gibbons et al., 2007; Gibbons and deGruy, 2019; Gibbons and Hedeker, 1992; Graham et al., 2006). The University of California, Los Angeles, uses CAT-MH to screen all its undergraduates for both overall assessment and to triage students for further care. A similar screening tool is offered by the American Foundation for Suicide Prevention. This online program[8] is being used by mental health services at institutions of higher education, including community colleges and undergraduate, graduate, medical, veterinary, and other professional programs. Individuals can anonymously communicate with the program's counselor to receive recommendations, feedback, and support for connecting to available mental health services.

INSTITUTIONAL CAPACITY TO PROVIDE NEEDED SERVICES

Once an institution has determined the extent of mental health and substance use issues among its students, there are four critical steps that follow: determining the scope of services needed to meet the measured demand; assessing what resources the institution has available on campus and in the community to meet that demand; assessing how existing resources are deployed and how effectively they are meeting mission objectives; and closing the gap between what is needed and what is available at the institution and in the community. Colleges and university budgets will constrain the scope of services available on campus, so each institution should evaluate the mixture of services available on campus, in the local community, and online—to support student wellbeing and provide care for those students in need. Institutions may decide to pay particular attention and allocate funding for specific types of treatment in the event there are no services available in the surrounding community.

The committee recognizes that the availability of financial and personnel resources to enact changes necessary to better meet students' wellbeing, mental health, and substance use treatment needs will likely be a major constraint, especially in the short term given the financial impact of the COVID-19 pandemic on institutional budgets. Nonetheless, the committee believes that institutions of higher education should give greater priority to addressing students' mental health, substance use, and wellbeing issues given that the stress of the pandemic, economic instability, and increasing social isolation will continue to affect students' lives. Institutional commitment and leadership are essential elements moving forward.

---

[8] Additional information is available at https://afsp.org/interactive-screening-program (accessed June 24, 2020).

Leadership from higher education is not enough, however. Moving forward successfully also depends on local, state, and federal policies that allocate resources and mandate the ways they should be utilized. Therefore, some of the solutions recommended here depend on policy changes at one or more levels of government. However, given that university leaders today are likely analyzing the use of resources in the face of the financial challenges wrought by the COVID-19 pandemic, the time is ripe for those leaders to include identifying resources and opportunities to improve the mental health and wellbeing of their students.

In the wake of COVID-19, the American Council of Education surveyed nearly 200 college and university presidents regarding their major concerns in response to the pandemic. The results from April 2020 indicated that 51 percent of university presidents already provide mental health services for their students and did not have the resources for additional support. Thirty-five percent stated that they have existing services and planned to invest more resources, while 12 percent stated that they do not currently offer clinical services, but are considering additional options to address student mental health and substance abuse in light of COVID-19 (Turk et al., 2020). This survey, which does not include community colleges and is not representative of the entire scope of this report, does reflect the reality that even in a global pandemic, 63 percent of the leaders surveyed recognized the need for resources; however, they did not necessarily have the means to increase clinical support.

In addition to these concerns, there are not enough mental health and substance use professionals in the country to meet the needs of the general population, with some regions experiencing greater shortages than others. In particular, there is a severe, nation-wide shortage of providers who are both participating providers with insurance plans and accepting new patients. Institutions of higher education often suffer from the same problem, lacking a sufficient number of mental health professionals to care for their student population. The Health Resources and Services Administration projected in 2016 that the supply of workers in mental health professions would be short by some 250,000 individuals by 2025 (Health Resources and Services Administration, 2016). Already in 2020, two-thirds of primary care physicians report having difficulty referring patients for mental health care, compared to roughly one-third for referrals to other specialties (Bishop et al., 2016).

Dealing with the Shortage of Mental Health and Substance Use Professionals

At the same time that there is a shortage of mental health and substance use professionals, demand for mental health and substance use services on college campuses has been rising steadily for several years (CCMH, 2017, 2020a) (see Box 5-5). As a result, institutions of higher education have been struggling to meet the rising demand for mental health and substance use services, which

---

BOX 5-5
The Clinical Load Index

According to the International Accreditation of Counseling Services (IACS), "every effort should be made to maintain minimum staffing ratios in the range of one fulltime equivalent professional staff member (excluding trainees) to every 1,000 to 1,500 students, depending on services offered and other campus mental health agencies" (IACS, 2019b). This guiding rationale, however, has become insufficient as a standard for many smaller institutions and unreachable for many large institutions (CCMH, 2020a). To create a more informative standard, CCMH developed the Clinical Load Index (CLI) (CCMH, 2020c) in partnership with IACS and AUCCCD, which describes the relationship between the supply of and demand for mental health services at colleges and universities. Instead of recommending a single score, the CLI provides institutions with a description of the range of staffing options and aims to describe the characteristics of various score-ranges so that institutions can focus on the type of service they want to deliver and then staff appropriately. According to CCMH, an individual CLI score can be thought of as either "clients per standardized counselor per year," or "standardized annual case load." Higher CLI scores are typically associated with centers that function more as crisis and referral operations and that provide minimal ongoing care and with larger institutions and counseling centers that serve more students. Counseling centers with low CLI scores tend to be at smaller institutions that serve a higher percentage of the student body, provide more traditional weekly counseling, and have fewer treatment limits. Higher CLI scores are associated with fewer appointments, spaced farther apart, and significantly less improvement in depression, anxiety, and general distress by students in treatment (CCMH, 2020a).

---

exceeds capacity in many institutions. (Thielking, 2017). In 2018, some 43 percent of the 571 college and university counseling centers surveyed by the AUCCCD increased the number of staff positions in counseling centers, while less than 9 percent lost staff positions (LeViness et al., 2018). However, more than half of the counseling centers reported having one or more positions turn over during the previous year, with institutions noting that "low staff salaries and problematic center work conditions were factors in a significant proportion of this turnover." (LeViness, 2018, p. 1).

The most direct approach for increasing capacity is to commit institutional funding for mental health and substance use services and hire more staff to deliver those services, including psychologists, psychiatrists, professional counselors, social workers, nurse practitioners, case managers, and physician assistants with experience in the area of mental health and substance use. However, increased hiring may not be a realistic solution for many colleges and universities to pursue given limited budgets, building space availability, and challenges in hiring qualified staff.

Bridging Campus and Community
Resources to Increase Capacity

Students who cannot get the treatment they need through on-campus centers are increasingly seeking to access community-based care, when it is available. However, institutions of higher education can further support these students by ensuring that mechanisms exist to strengthen both treatment capacity in the community and continuity of care when students are referred off campus so that they do not fail to access care. One example is McLean Hospital's College Mental Health Program. This program "bridges the gap between a psychiatric hospital and multiple campus settings in an attempt to address the specific needs of college student-patients across levels of psychiatric care and diagnostic areas/programs," (Pinder-Amaker and Bell, 2012, p. 174). It also addresses a barrier that exists for many institutions, in that they may not know what resources exist in their communities or may not have arrangements with community mental health and substance use treatment resources to serve their students in need.

The problem of insufficient capacity is particularly acute at the nation's community colleges, where counselor to student ratios are nearly half those of baccalaureate degree-granting colleges. According to the Steve Fund, only 10 percent of community college students, at most, use on-campus mental health and substance use services (Primm, 2019). A survey of community colleges and four-year institutions in California found that community college students had more severe mental health concerns and fewer on-campus mental health resources than four-year college students (Katz and Davison, 2014). Some rural communities also face challenges related to health care broadly, with limited access to hospitals, specialty providers, and mental health services in their region (Kirby et al., 2019; O'Hanlon et al., 2019).

If an institution relies on community-based treatment options to help meet its students' demand for services, it should promote mechanisms to match students to community resources and enable them to use those resources easily, rather than leave students on their own to find and access community resources. There are several for-profit vendors of referral programs that can match students to community providers, as well as provide health and wellness services. Therapy for Black Girls, for example, is a free online service that aims to both reduce the stigma of treatment and help African American women, including students, find local community-based therapists. In 2019, the American College Health Association issued guidelines for institutions that are thinking of turning to outsourcing to student health needs[9] (ACHA, 2019c).

While outsourcing can in some cases provide students with access to a wider range of specialists and more highly trained staff, there are a number of potential disadvantages to outsourcing mental health services that institutions need to

---

[9] Available at: https://www.acha.org/documents/resources/guidelines/ACHA_Outsourcing_College_Health_Programs_May2019.pdf (accessed September 20, 2020).

consider in moving forward with this approach to expanding capacity (ACCA, 2020), including:

- An excessive focus on psychopathology at these services rather than modalities more appropriate for stress-inducing developmental challenges that colleges students often face.
- Possible session limits that may fail to produce significant clinical improvements.
- Students having to bear financial responsibility for services resulting from limits on insurance coverage.
- Reduced ability for students to network with student affairs and residence life staff.
- Potential reduction in outreach efforts and educational programming on the part of the institution that may promote mental health and prompt students to use on-campus counseling services.
- Reduced responsiveness of the institution to on-campus emergency situations, particularly those warranting immediate personal interventions when there are threats to self or others.

Using Telehealth to Increase Access

In addition to increasing connections to local providers, another method to increase students' access to mental health and substance use services is via telehealth and internet-based psychotherapy treatment programs (Berger, Boettcher, and Caspar, 2011, 2014; Kraepelien et al., 2019; Păsărelu et al., 2017). Notably, the COVID-19 pandemic has forced therapists and their clients to adopt this model during a time of widespread social distancing. This sudden transition has not always gone smoothly, but it does present an opportunity to identify best practices.

The Higher Education Mental Health Alliance has produced a guide to telehealth that outlines the potential benefits, limitations, and legal and ethical concerns regarding such services (Higher Education Mental Health Alliance, 2014), and the American Psychological Association has published guidelines for providing telepsychology services (JTFDTGP, 2013). Additionally, the American Psychiatric Association has developed best practice recommendations and identified special considerations for college students around the use of telehealth during the pandemic (American Psychiatric Association, APA Committee on Telepsychiatry & APA College Mental Health Caucus, 2020). Telehealth may on the one hand broaden access to services but can also pose equity concerns if all students do not have equal access to reliable broadband services. In addition, there is likely to be significant variability in the competence of psychotherapists to conduct telehealth sessions. Moreover, the effectiveness of telehealth across the broad range of mental health and substance use issues has not been studied in anywhere near the level of detail that traditional therapy has been. This suggests that some caution is appropriate in too widely recommending a telehealth approach.

On the other hand, expanding the use of internet-based therapeutic programs could provide an option that many students, including students of color and those from underrepresented populations, may prefer over face-to-face counseling. Tele-mental health approaches may also be particularly useful for rural or small colleges or for community colleges, where students may lack transportation to reach off-campus sites or where the distance to the nearest provider might be too far to travel. Additionally, by making specific forms of behaviorally focused mental health services readily available within the primary care setting, psychiatric consultation through telehealth to primary health care providers can serve as a mechanism to improve access. Using telehealth, the potential pool of therapists to refer to can potentially be state-wide, rather than limited to the local community. As institutions build capacity for care via telehealth and other internet-based services, it will be important to conduct ongoing assessments of outcomes and experiences.

The Imperative to Provide Equitable Support to Students of All Identities

As colleges and universities work to determine how to increase mental health services, leadership should ensure that the personnel, resources, and programs are inclusive of the identities of individuals represented on the campus and historically underrepresented in academia. Programs should review the use of language, images, and examples to decrease bias, reduce harm, and to ensure representation. Exclusionary language and imagery can pose harm to students' sense of belonging, harm their mental health, and create a sense of alienation from others on campus. For non-binary students and students who are sexual and gender minorities, forms that limit gender selection to "female" and "male," for example, suggests that their gender identity does not exist or is not important enough for recognition.

In the absence of such intentionality, some solutions might exacerbate mental health care disparities by further marginalizing those who may experience particularly high levels of stigma related to health-seeking behavior. Studies have found that the stigma around mental health and substance use treatment services is particularly high among students of color (Cheng, Kawn, and Sevig, 2013; Lipson et al., 2018; Liu et al., 2019a). Additionally, feelings of marginalization and isolation appear to be experienced at higher rates by BIPOC and SGM students (Cabral and Smith, 2011; NASEM, 2016; Wilson and Cariola, 2019). It is worth noting that COVID-19 may exacerbate the existing gap in health inequalities mentioned above. Students from these groups may also experience higher rates of stress related to disproportionately high infection rates and deaths among BIPOC communities.

The Center for Applied Research Solutions has developed a guide, trainings, and technical assistance for supporting students from diverse racial and ethnic backgrounds enrolled at California's community colleges.[10] This and the Equity in Mental Health Framework, discussed above, are resources that can serve as the foundation and as guides for colleges and universities, assisting them in creating more specific strategies to ensure service to the students on each campus.

Peer-to-peer support initiatives may be helpful in many ways for students of color, particularly when facilitated by a mental health liaison (Naslund et al., 2016). Research has shown that young people with personal and emotional problems and individuals from historically excluded communities are more likely to seek help from their friends and family than from other sources, including mental health professionals (Barker, Olukoya, and Aggleton, 2005; Offer et al., 1991). For international students, peer support may provide community and a sense of connection and may serve as a guide to understanding unfamiliar customs and social norms. In addition, graduate students with strong support from peers are significantly less likely to screen positively for anxiety and depression (Posselt, 2020). Whether and how a peer responds to someone developing mental health problems or who is in a crisis situation can make a difference as to whether appropriate professional help is received. The 12-hour Mental Health First Aid course[11] (Kitchener, Jorm, and Kelly, 2017) is specifically designed to train people, including young adults, to provide appropriate help to a person developing a mental health problem or in a mental health crisis (Hadlaczky et al., 2014; Jorm et al., 2019). Peer-to-peer initiatives are powerful not only in building a support system, but also at a more fundamental level, raising students' knowledge and awareness of these issues and how they play out within their own campus communities (Sontag-Padilla et al., 2018a). However, it is critical to recognize that a consequence of programs designed to raise awareness and empower community members to refer students of concern, is likely to be increased demand for mental health services. Therefore, when considering the implementation of programs such as these, institutions should be prepared for subsequently addressing a growth in demand for services.

Making appropriate mental health services more available in primary care settings can also facilitate students' access to mental health care and improve coordination between mental health and primary care providers, both on campus and in telehealth services. While some forms of mental health care should be considered for integration with primary care, institutions should also recognize that mental health care is a highly specialized field of independent practice that can exist independently of the primary care environment.

---

[10] Additional information is available at http://cccstudentmentalhealth.org/docs/SMHP-Diverse-Racial-Ethnic-Students.pdf (accessed April 27, 2020).

[11] Additional information is available at https://www.mentalhealthfirstaid.org/take-a-course (accessed June 24, 2020).

RECOMMENDATION 5-7
Institutions of higher education should work to ensure students have access to high-quality mental health and substance use treatment services. These services can be provided either on campus or in the local community. In order to ensure students have this access:

- After conducting a needs assessment and reviewing available mental health resources on and off campus, institutional leadership should attempt to measure and define the "gap" between need for mental health care and capacity for care. That gap should then be examined for solutions from multiple angles but especially long-term funding strategies and/or community partnerships.
- Institutions of higher education should design and implement culturally responsive services and programs to serve the needs and identities of all students.
- Colleges and universities should make behaviorally focused mental health services more readily available in primary care settings to facilitate students' access to care and improve coordination between mental health and primary care providers, both on campus and in telehealth services.
- Institutions of higher education should create collaborative relationships in the community that will increase clinician diversity to better serve diverse student populations.
- If counseling centers rely on community-based resources to meet the mental health needs of their students, they should consider investing in case managers/resource navigators to help students connect with these community-based resources.
- Institutions can make wide use of telehealth options for those populations and situations for which it is appropriate.

DEVELOPING FACULTY, STAFF, AND STUDENT CAPABILITY TO SUPPORT EMOTIONAL WELLBEING AND MENTAL HEALTH

As noted in the introduction to this chapter, it takes everyone on campus to contribute to an environment that fosters student wellbeing, helps protect students from developing mental health and substance use issues, and helps facilitate students' access to services that would benefit them. All those who are in regular contact with students have an important role in this effort. At some institutions, particularly community colleges, faculty are likely to be the only staff members with whom students interact on a regular basis. Faculty-student interactions are also a critical factor in student persistence to program completion and graduation (Boone et al., 2020; Lillis, 2011; Wirt and Jaeger, 2014), and the quality of support from faculty is clearly related to student wellbeing (Baik, Lacombe, and Brooker, 2019; Posselt, 2018a).

However, one result of the narrow focus of current training in Ph.D. programs[12]—the primary training ground for faculty—is that most faculty have not received any formal training to help them create student-oriented learning and research environments where a diverse set of students will thrive (Posselt, 2020). To the contrary, the classroom and lab can be sites in which students experience discrimination, harassment, even assault—often on the basis of marginalized social identities (Lane, 2016; Rojas-Sosa, 2016; Wadsworth, Hecht, and Jung, 2008). At the same time, a major factor contributing to high graduate student attrition rates is a poor relationship with a research advisor, with neglect, exploitation, and even abuse being common complaints, particularly from students from underrepresented populations (Brunsma, Embrick, and Shin, 2016; Curtin et al., 2013; Ong et al., 2011; Spalter-Roth and Erskine, 2007).

Much like the broad diversity and inclusion considerations discussed in the National Academies report *Graduate STEM Education for the 21st Century* (NASEM, 2018a), the culture of many institutions of higher education and their incentive structures—at both the disciplinary level as well as tenure and promotion within instiutions—have been poorly aligned with creating inclusive environments. Many doctoral students working in the arts and humanities experience isolation and may not have regular meetings with their research advisors. On the other hand, individuals in lab-based programs who share equipment and facilities may encounter interpersonal tensions with other members of the lab or face different challenges working with a principal investigator. Work environments matter greatly for creating a culture of wellbeing (Levecque et al., 2017).

Faculty Can Help Address Student Mental Health Issues

There are several ways in which faculty can help students deal with mental health and substance use issues without directly providing counseling or other treatment services themselves. Most faculty, however, are unaware they can help. Even if they do know this, few faculty have received the training needed to identify problems, refer students for help, and provide students with the means to bolster their wellbeing on their own. Some faculty also have concerns about possible liability issues associated with getting involved. The committee stresses that faculty and staff should not be trained to provide therapy themselves and staff or act in the place of licensed mental health care providers. Instead, faculty and staff should focus on designing learning environments and adopting behaviors that prioritize student learning, emphasize wellbeing, and recognize early signs of distress in students.

Doing so is not impossible—the Healthy Universities program in the United Kingdom (Newton, Dooris, and Wills, 2016) and Australia's Enhancing University

---

[12] Ph.D. programs focus heavily on the development of research expertise to the neglect of knowledge and skills for managing instruction, people, and projects. The National Academies have recommended that these skills be added to all graduate training programs (NASEM, 2018a).

Student project,[13] for example, are working to do so and could serve as examples for U.S. institutions of higher education to follow. Closer to home, the University of Texas at Austin's unique Wellbeing in Learning Environments program "helps faculty make small shifts in teaching that could make a major difference in students' mental health and wellbeing" (University of Texas at Austin, 2019). The National Association of State Mental Health Program Directors (NASMHPD) has issued a guide for staff and administrators that offers advice on recognizing signs and effectively engaging and accommodating students with mental health problems (Jones, Bower, Furuzawa, 2016a). The REDFLAGS model, which has been shown to have utility in community and four-year colleges, is one approach that gives faculty a simple mechanism to flag possible mental health or substance use problems (Kalkbrenner and Carlisle, 2019; Kalkbrenner et al., 2019).

The Red Folder at Penn State University[14] is another method of sharing resources and providing support to faculty, staff, graduate student instructors, postdoctoral researchers, and others who work with students. Penn State designed this resource as a reference guide to recognize, respond effectively to, and refer distressed students for care (Penn State Red Folder). The Red Folder is a physical object, in addition to an online resource, that can serve as a quick reference with resources related to academic, psychological, physical, and safety-risk issues. The University of California also has a Red Folder Initiative,[15] which provides customized information about common signs of student distress. The counseling center provides a brief training on the folder that includes guidance on emergency contacts, follow-up tips, and how to connect students with the most appropriate resources (UCOP Red Folder). Though the efforts described above are rooted in knowledge from peer-reviewed research, evaluations of these efforts that account for the diverse experiences of students from different demographic groups and in different institutional contexts will be important for understanding the efficacy of these approaches in supporting student mental health.

In addition to identifying students in need and referring them to campus resources, faculty can support student mental health by taking steps to design learning environments that prioritize student learning and wellbeing (see Box 5-6 for an example of a program promoting student wellbeing at the University of Texas at Austin). For example, faculty can make use of the resources provided by the Universal Design for Learning framework, which offers guidance on how "to improve and optimize teaching and learning for all people based on scientific insights into how humans learn."[16] Among the guidance offered by this framework

---

[13] Additional information is available at http://unistudentwellbeing.edu.au/framework (accessed April 30, 2020).

[14] Additional information is available at https://redfolder.psu.edu/ (accessed August 26, 2020).

[15] Additional information is available at https://www.ucop.edu/student-mental-health-resources/training-and-programs/faculty-and-staff-outreach/red-folder-initiative.html (accessed August 26, 2020).

[16] Additional information is available at http://udlguidelines.cast.org (accessed November 12, 2020).

BOX 5-6
Wellbeing in Learning Environments Program
University of Texas at Austin

Like many universities, UT Austin has found a growing demand for mental health services among its students. The university reports that the demand for mental health services increased 88 percent from academic year 2009-2010 to academic year 2018-2019, while the total number of students at The University of Texas at Austin increased by 1.6 percent (CMHC Fact Sheet, 2019; UT Austin, 2020). Further, UT Austin found that students indicated, "that faculty members are often seen as the 'missing link' when it comes to their own well-being (Stuart and Lee, 2013)." In response to this issue, the university developed its Well-being in Learning Environments program, which offers faculty a guidebook with a variety of strategies—based in research and the experiences of fellow UT Austin faculty—to use in the classroom to support student wellbeing. The guidebook advises faculty to "pick and choose" approaches that best fit with their interpersonal and teaching style and offers the following advice on how to promote general wellbeing:

- On the first day of class, use a survey to get to know students. Ask about their backgrounds, interests, strengths, needs, and other topics.
- Share personal connections to content—areas where you struggled, concepts you were surprised to learn, etc.
- Let students see you make mistakes, then show them how you use those mistakes to learn.
- Struggle with concepts in front of students and allow them to help you work through the process.
- Focus less on competition and performance and more on learning and mastery. For example, allowing students to retake exams or parts of exams to learn from mistakes.
- Share ways that you practice self-care, and have students share how they practice it as well.
- Include information in your syllabus about mental health (but avoid copying and pasting this information from somewhere else).
- Talk about mental health openly to destigmatize it.
- Let students know you are open to talking with them individually about their states of well-being.
- Provide a "mindfulness minute" at the beginning of class, before exams, etc., in which you encourage or allow students to sit quietly and use deep breathing techniques.
- Be flexible. Take into consideration students' lives outside of class.

The guide goes on to offer faculty specific practices they can adopt to promote social connectedness, mindfulness, growth mindset, resilience, gratitude, inclusivity, self-compassion, empathy, and life purpose.

Source: https://www.cmhc.utexas.edu/wellbeing/images/guidebook.pdf.

are strategies for (1) reducing threats and distractions that can undermine learning and (2) identifying pedagogical approaches that contribute to student stress. For example, research has shown that some approaches to active learning exercises in STEM classes can lead to student anxiety (Cooper et al. 2018).

Faculty can also support student wellbeing through effective mentoring; however, institutions of higher education, with few exceptions, have left mentoring to happen organically or on an ad hoc basis, as was noted in the 2019 NASEM report *The Science of Effective Mentorship in STEMM* (NASEM, 2019b). As that report details, good mentorship is an acquired skill and faculty and staff can learn the skills they need to become good, supportive mentors. The Entering Mentoring curriculum, for example, has been used to educate thousands of mentors in the United States (Pfund, Brandchaw, and Handelsman, 2015).

Taken together, what the committee envisions is an approach that would provide faculty with basic training in four areas:

1. how to identify, initiate conversations with, and refer to treatment those students who may be having problems with mental health or substance use
2. how to make learning environments inclusive and supportive of student wellbeing
3. how to model preventive strategies and coping skills in class
4. how to improve mentorship and pedagogical skills so that relationships and instruction support wellbeing.

To involve faculty more directly in efforts to address student mental health, faculty will require adequate support, including training, from the institution. For example, it is well documented that women and faculty of color bear a disproportionate burden of providing mentoring and student support, which extends to supporting student mental health. Therefore, there is a need to ensure that the responsibility and time for supporting students is equally distributed across faculty. To this end, faculty should be expected to and be rewarded for supporting students in this manner, including through formal evaluation processes such as tenure and promotion.

In line with recommendations from a recent NASEM (2020) report that examined promising practices for addressing the underrepresentation of women in STEMM, academia should similarly take steps to formally recognize, support, and reward efforts toward enhancing student wellbeing for faculty members, as well as those counseling staff who have taken on more of the service burden. Promoting student mental health is everyone's responsibility to the extent possible.

RECOMMENDATION 5-8
Provide and require faculty training on how to create an inclusive and healthy learning environment.
- Provide and require faculty training about how to recognize students in distress and appropriately refer them to appropriate care.
- Provide mentor training, starting in graduate school, for all faculty, recognizing that good mentorship practices serve as a protective factor for student mental health.

Raising Mental Health and Suicide Awareness

In addition to developing capacity to address student mental health and substance use issues, institutions of higher education must take several other steps to benefit their students (Travia et al., 2019). The first is to reduce the stigma associated with seeking help for mental health and substance use issues. The California Community Colleges, for example, have used a suite of six online, interactive training simulations from Kognito, a for-profit entity, to reduce stigma and engage faculty, staff, and students in supporting those exhibiting signs of distress. The result was a 73 percent increase in the number of students that faculty, staff, and students referred to mental health services across 113 campuses (Kognito, 2016; Sontag-Padilla et al., 2018c). Other campuses have developed websites listing all available mental health and substance use resources on campus and in the community or used posters around campus alerting students how to access help if they are suicidal or otherwise suffering emotionally. This type of intervention would help to better align interventions designed to increase referrals with growing service capacity to accommodate increased referrals.

Institutions of higher education can also help prevent suicide, the second leading cause of death among U.S. college and university students (Liu et al., 2019; Turner, Leno, and Keller, 2013). Researchers suggests that "preventing suicide on college campuses requires a systemic approach supported by broad campus-wide cooperation. Students who die by or attempt suicide typically do not seek professional help before doing so, making outreach, faculty and staff training, and good referral systems even more critical" (Brownson et al., 2011, 2014). A comprehensive approach to suicide prevention includes promoting social networks and connectedness, improving access to mental health services on and off campus, identifying and assisting students who may be a risk for suicide, and being prepared to respond when a suicide death occurs (SPRC, 2020). These strategies, in conjunction with the policies and procedures that support them, are what constitute a campus-wide suicide prevention plan. Ideally, such a plan is embedded in policies throughout the college that are part of a larger plan to support student wellbeing. Numerous organizations have developed guides to help colleges and universities develop suicide prevention programs (JED Foundation and EDC, 2011; SPRC, 2004).

Along these lines, many institutions have established behavior intervention teams[17] (HEMHA, 2012; JED Foundation, 2013). According to the JED Foundation, these teams "promote student, faculty, and staff success and campus safety by facilitating the identification and support of individuals who demonstrate behaviors that may be early warning signs of possible troubled, disruptive, or violent behavior" (Jed Foundation, 2016).

The main reason colleges and universities establish such teams is to "provide a mechanism for improved coordination and communication across a campus or system, especially when various departments are perceived to be or are actually operating in their own silos" (HEMHA, 2012, p. 3). Areas of concern, according to the Higher Education Mental Health Alliance's guide for such teams, include psychosocial and mental problems that may "both interfere with adequate and successful functioning that, if unaddressed, might lead to a dangerous outcome to the student or the community" (HEMHA, 2012, p. 4). The appeal of this approach is the possibility of identifying problems and intervening before they become potentially dangerous (see Chapter 4 for more information about campus response to student death by suicide).

Account for the Importance of Communities in Shaping Student Wellbeing

Research has shown that communities, not solely individuals, shape health, and college and university communities are no exception (Slusser et al., 2018; Sontag-Padilla et al., 2018b; Weil, 2014). The healthy campus movement, ongoing at numerous institutions of higher education, is built on efforts to engage the entire campus population of students, staff, and faculty in building physical and mental health and wellbeing into a college or university's culture.[18] Examples of programs under way include Healthy CUNY at City College of New York, the University of California, Los Angeles's Health Campus Initiative, Duke University's DukeReach, The University of Texas at Austin's Wellness Network, the integrated health and wellness program at Jefferson Community College in rural New York, Dartmouth College's Mentoring with Purpose Program, and The University of Wisconsin-Superior's Pruitt Center for Mindfulness and Wellbeing. National efforts are also taking hold, such as those promoted by Active Minds, the National Center on Safe Supportive Learning Environments, Healthier America, and Bringing Theory to Practice. The Gallup Organization even offers a "Wellbeing University Certification" that provides a tailored strategy to promote campus

---

[17] The focus of Behavioral Intervention Teams varies. Some campuses have one team that covers all issues, while others have specific teams for emergencies and threat management.

[18] Additional information is available at https://www.acha.org/HealthyCampus/Implement/MAP-IT_Framework/HealthyCampus/Map-It_Framework.aspx?hkey=bc5a1b28-ae96-4f06-b3ee-ed-492441e7db (accessed April 28, 2020).

wellbeing.[19] The common feature of all of these initiatives is that they recognize that institutions of higher education have the capacity to infuse health and wellbeing into their campus cultures, but only with the support and engagement of all of the siloed interests and communities that exist on campus.

Provide All Students with Formal Instruction on How to Develop and Maintain Wellbeing

One suggestion the committee received during its information-gathering activities was for institutions to develop a course for all entering students, graduate students, and professional students that teaches them how to maintain wellbeing, continually aspire toward being well, and overcome the inevitable challenges they will experience both in college and in life. It is not clear that an entire, semester-long course is required, but it is the committee's judgment that every student should receive some formal education or training on the concept of wellbeing and how they might maintain it in the context of the pressures surrounding higher education. The issues may differ based on the program level (undergraduate, graduate, and professional) and could include custom features to address specific program elements, such as thesis work, field or off-site research, or comprehensive exams. This training, which might be deliverable through a web-based program (Ahmad et al., 2020), could also inform students as to what they should do when experiencing a mental health or substance use problem.

NASMHPD has a free toolkit for students who have received treatment for early mental health issues that offers specific modules with concrete advice on how best to obtain support on campus and thrive in their pursuit of higher education (Jones, Bower, and Furuzawa, 2016b). Other resources include *Becoming a Master Student* (Ellis, 2017), which provides diverse information focusing on whole-person development, and Kognito, which offers online student mental health workshops that engage students in role-play conversations with virtual humans. Kognito's simulations have been used with Native Americans (Bartgis and Albright, 2016), Latinx students (Albright, 2018), veterans (Albright and McMillan, 2018), and SGM students (Marshall, 2016). It is important to note that there are many non- and for-profit entities entering the virtual space around mental health, and not all of the services have been created based on evidence (see Chapter 2 for additional information).

Institutions, including medical schools (Slavin, 2018, 2019; Slavin, Schindler, and Chibnall, 2014) and community colleges (Cuseo, 1997), that offer such courses have found they help promote a healthy transition to the institution (Choate and Smith, 2003; Ellis, 2017; Lockwood and Wohl, 2012). For example, Choate and Smith found that "the infusion of a wellness model into the

---

[19] Additional information is available at https://www.gallup.com/education/194297/student-life-outcomes-matter.aspx (accessed June 15, 2020).

curriculum of a required orientation course for first-year students was related to changes in student wellness," as measured by a "quantitative analysis of student WEL score profiles and an analysis of students' written reflections." Students reported "that the wellness model enhanced their learning through increasing self-awareness, self-direction, recognition of the interrelatedness of all life areas, the identification of strengths and areas for improvement, and appreciation for the specific application of strategies for change" and demonstrated improvements in target areas for improvement, according to their WEL score profile, in areas such as stress management and nutrition (Choate and Smith, 2003). Similarly, Lockwood and Wohl found that "a lifetime wellness course can improve physical self-efficacy and promote changes in wellness behaviors, especially in the area of physical wellness" for students (Lockwood and Wohl, 2012).

An additional important role these courses play is to raise awareness about the resources available for students in need (Canby et al., 2015; Conley, Travers, and Bryant, 2013; Dvořáková et al., 2017; Parcover et al., 2018; Stephens, Hamedani, and Destin, 2014; Walton and Cohen, 2011). Such a class could also serve as a community-building activity that engages students in efforts to create a wellbeing-supporting culture across campus. Consistent with other recommendations, institutions should be aware that courses like these are likely to increase the demand for mental health and substance use services as a natural consequence of raising awareness of those services. Without education and raising student awareness, simply increasing access to services will not suffice.

RECOMMENDATION 5-9
As a part of formal orientation to college life, all students should participate in structured opportunities to learn about individual wellbeing and the cultivation of a healthy, respectful campus climate. This orientation should also include material on how to develop resilience in the face of inevitable challenges they will experience both in college and in life.

- To enable students' self-awareness and resilience, training should acknowledge how behaviors such as sleep, nutrition, exercise, social media, and work can be both levers for wellbeing as well as affected by wellbeing.
- Training should also include information on how to recognize and address implicit bias, and about the essential role students themselves play in creating a community that supports each other's wellbeing.
- Each institution should also periodically offer refresher or "booster" training on these issues.
- Institutions should regularly and widely provide guidance to students and faculty on mental health resources available on campus and in the community.

RECOMMENDATION 5-10

Institutions of higher education should recognize that there is no single approach to promoting wellbeing and dealing with mental health and substance use problems that will be appropriate to all student populations.

- Support services should be tailored to the unique histories, circumstances, and needs of individual student populations.
- Support services should recognize and respond to the fact that many students from diverse populations will have experienced interpersonal racism, systemic racism, and implicit bias both before and during their time in higher education.

6

A Research Agenda

From the outset of this project, it has been clear to the committee that determining how best to deliver mental health, substance use, and wellbeing services to the wide variety of students enrolled at the nation's diverse array of institutions of higher education is an area badly in need of rigorous, theory-based research. What follows in this chapter are some of the key areas of research that the committee believes would help institutions of higher education better prepare for and provide mental health and substance use interventions and create environments that better support student wellbeing.

DEVELOPING, EVALUATING, AND SUSTAINING A CAMPUS CULTURE CENTERED IN WELLBEING

At the broadest level of public health and wellbeing programs and approaches, there is limited research to guide colleges and universities on ways to ensure that the entire campus, including virtual spaces, promotes wellbeing. This can vary from different definitions of wellbeing and how priorities may shift based on student demographics. Regarding institutional culture change, there is already a substantial body of research pertaining to culture change in and benefits to corporate and health care environments (Alvesson and Sveningsson, 2016; Bendak, Shikhli, and Abdel-Razek, 2020; Carlson et al., 2016; Choi, Oh, and Colbert, 2015; Edmondson and Lei, 2014; Parmelli et al., 2011). There is a need, however, to extend those type of studies to the academic environment.

- What is wellbeing in the context of institutions of higher education? Of different types of institutions?

- How can wellbeing be measured, both for the individual student and across the entire campus? What public health approaches can be used to embed a culture of wellbeing?
- What approaches will work for transmitting the concept of wellbeing across the campus, including in hybrid and virtual settings? How do approaches differ by role on campus (student, faculty, administration, and beyond)? Through rigorous trials, what could we learn about the factors and components that are needed to deliver seminars, workshops, and other training related to wellbeing?
- How effective are faculty and mentor training opportunities in shifting their mindsets and behaviors with respect to serving students? What elements or processes of professional development are most impactful?
- What approaches work for improving well-being for students who are BIPOC and from historically excluded groups? What would be the best ways to tailor those approaches to the different subpopulations of students?
- For colleges and universities that have limited community resources related to wellbeing or to enact new programs, are there approaches that have a lower cost burden? What is the current availability of existing wellness resources for students?
- Do programs that institutions of higher education have implemented to address student wellbeing in fact improve student mental health?
- Can virtual programs and mobile applications support student wellbeing and mental health? What are their limitations and appropriate uses? How can research inform strategies to increase engagement of students with digital health programs to address the fact that programs are only effective when people engage at a meaningful level, which is challenging with young people online?
- What is the impact of peer support programs on student wellbeing, mental health, and substance use?
- In terms of safety, privacy, and ethical use of social media, what training and education can colleges provide students so that they understand their rights and the risks involved?
- In the event there is a death of a student by suicide, what are the best ways to share information about the student while respecting the rights of the family and providing additional support to those who have been affected by the death?
- Trauma has interpersonal and cognitive consequences that advances in screening and evaluation are increasingly able to document and measure. Screenings also increase the understanding of the relationship between trauma and behavioral outcomes in terms of substance use, attention, self-regulation, and stress management, as well as one's ability to access to higher-order skills necessary for academic success such as abstract thinking and problem solving. As much of the existing

research exists in the youth and K-12 space, how can additional research understand the impact of trauma and how to support students with trauma to and through higher education?

Factors That Affect Student Mental Health, Substance Use, and Wellbeing

The available evidence suggests that the campus environment has unique characteristics that affect student mental health and wellbeing. Some of these are risk factors, such as widespread substance use, and others are protective factors, such as likelihood of being from a higher socioeconomic status than age-matched students not enrolled in higher education. Additionally, understanding which factors impact students prior to their arrival on campus may give campuses the ability to market their services and increase visibility to those who could benefit the most from a suite of wellbeing as well as other academic services. The ability to understand the factors that impact students during the time they are enrolled, including how factors may change based on their setting (in-person, hybrid, or online learning, or being primarily off campus for research), could enable institutions to amplify beneficial factors and work to reduce or eliminate detrimental factors. Answers to these questions would greatly help colleges and universities adjust their services.

- How has the COVID-19 pandemic affected the wellbeing and mental health of students?
- What is the link between student wellbeing and educational outcomes?
- What are the long-term consequences of remote/virtual learning on student mental health and wellbeing? The long-term impacts of COVID on the college experience should be studied over time.
- What risk and protective factors in the campus environment impact undergraduate and graduate student mental health, substance use, and wellbeing?
- What role does prior or current exposure to trauma play in student wellbeing and mental health?
- What are productive and effective ways to engage families in addressing student issues of mental health, substance use, and wellbeing?
- What role does injury (including traumatic brain injury, etc.) resulting from sports and/or combat exposure among veterans play in student wellbeing and mental health?
- What roles do post-graduate stressors play in student wellbeing and mental health?
- What roles do individual and cognitive factors play in student wellbeing and mental health?
- What roles do the social and environmental determinants of health play in student wellbeing and mental health?

- What is the comorbidity between mental health and substance use, and how does comorbidity affect treatment outcomes?
- How has the increase in vaping tobacco products affected student mental health?
- What changes have states that have changed laws around marijuana use (legalization and decriminalization) seen in the student and non-student population? How have use rates correlated with other health outcomes? Are there new public health, prevention, addiction, and recovery services in these states?
- What can predominantly white institutions learn from Minority Serving Institutions (MSIs) with respect to wellbeing of students who are BIPOC?

POLICIES THAT PROMOTE POSITIVE STUDENT MENTAL HEALTH AND WELLBEING AND LOW LEVELS OF SUBSTANCE USE

The impact of federal, state, and local regulations related to higher education policies would benefit from additional research to determine whether they are having the desired impacts and whether they might be at risk for harming students.

- How do policies related to health leave impact students? Do the policies comply with the Americans with Disabilities Act? What are the best approaches in terms of providing guidance to students, ongoing support when students are on leave, and return to campus? What student outcomes and experiences are associated with different admission and mental health leave of absence policies? How does this vary between undergraduate and graduate students?
- Are there ways, beyond the updated joint guidance document the Department of Education issued in December 2019,[1] to provide clearer guidance to colleges and universities regarding management of student treatment records and compliance with federal regulations such as Family Educational Rights and Privacy Act and Health Insurance Portability and Accountability Act ? How can colleges and universities providing services to students based on the ADA and Title IX do so with clarity and support in mind, rather than with compliance as the driving factor?
- How has higher education used local, state, and federal programs to address student insecurities regarding basic needs such as food and housing insecurity? Are there ways for more partnerships to ensure basic provisions for students?
- How can policymakers better understand and address the issues caused by state-specific licensing and the boundaries created? How can policymakers

---

[1] Available at https://studentprivacy.ed.gov/resources/joint-guidance-application-ferpa-and-hipaa-student-health-records (accessed September 23, 2020).

address barriers to providing effective telehealth, including across state lines? Are there ways that lawmakers can evaluate the impact of the temporary waivers granted during COVID-19 and ensure that effective measures are continued?

- How can campus leadership improve how they use research evidence to inform their decisions about programs and policies?
- What are the impacts of federal, state, and local investments on student mental health, substance use, and wellbeing? What are the academic and lifelong impacts of these investments?
- What are the impacts of federal and state policies on the resources, services, and outcomes for MSIs, notably historically designated Historically Black Colleges and Universities and Tribal Colleges and Universities ? Are there ways to understand federal and state policies related to higher education and the impacts on MSIs?
- How can more providers gain evidence-based training, education, licensure, and ongoing professional development to serve the needs of students?

Mental Health, Substance Use, and Wellbeing Collaborations between Higher Education and Community Providers

The earlier chapters of the report include recommendations that encourage campuses to commit extensive energy and resources to raising awareness of the offices, programs, and scope of care so that students know where to seek services where they are in need and know the level of care available. Students also have a responsibility before arriving to campus to gain a broad understanding of the health, wellbeing, and academic support services available to them. As the report states, there is a tension that colleges and universities must tread in the provision of mental health, substance use, and wellbeing services. Overall, the state of health and mental health care in the United States is limited in terms of providers that take insurance, the cost of copays, the availability of mental health specialists, and the availability of providers within a given area. In addition, higher education institutions have seen cuts in their budgets overall throughout recent decades. This means that students seeking services are looking to two systems, higher education and the U.S. medical system, that have may not have the resources students need. Addressing the U.S. mental health care system was out of the scope of this report; however, additional research for leaders in higher education to develop appropriate partnerships with community providers would be useful.

- What is the role of local hospitals and providers providing mental health services to the student population?
- What are the ways in which colleges and universities can receive reimbursement from health insurance companies for their provision of health care services to students?

- What is the most effective way to provide mental health services to specific populations of students, including, but not limited to:
  - Black, Indigenous, and people of color (BIPOC)
  - Students with disabilities and disabled students
  - First-generation students
  - International students and students without documentation
  - Student-athletes
  - Graduate students
  - Medical and other professional school students (e.g., nursing, pharmacy)
  - Post-traditional and non-traditional students
  - Sexual and gender minorities
  - Student survivors of trauma
  - Student military service members and veterans
- How can trauma-informed frameworks be integrated into other functional areas within higher education (e.g., teaching, mentoring, communications)? What are the outcomes?
- In terms of trauma-informed care for survivors of sexual assault and harassment, how can additional research provide more information around the sexual harassment experiences of women who are BIPOC and from other historically excluded groups? What kinds of policies, procedures, trainings, and interventions can prevent sexually harassing behavior, decrease the perceived organizational tolerance for sexually harassing behavior, and reduce harm to those who report incidents? How can organizations provide protection to those who experience sexually harassing behavior, associated retaliation, and the impact of harassment in the ambient environment?
- How should institutions of higher education best provide recovery programs for students returning to campus after a leave of absence?
- What is the impact of policies and programs initiated to support student wellbeing and mental health during the COVID-19 pandemic?
- In what ways can telehealth and virtual therapy provide evidence-based, high-quality mental health services in the higher education environment? Are there differential outcomes across student groups and for students with different concerns or problems?
- How effective and efficient are alternative strategies for implementing tiered systems of care, such as triaging, identifying needs, and filtering and engaging with appropriate level of care? Are there settings or groups of students where these strategies are more effective?

Addressing the Limited Data and Research Related to Mental Health, Substance Use, and Wellbeing in Higher Education

One of the major challenges noted across the report is the limited data related to these issues in a higher education setting. In addition to the broad challenges, there are certain types of institutions that have greater data gaps such as HBCUs, TCUs, and community colleges. There are also groups that would benefit from datasets that have greater capacity for disaggregation across a number of dimensions. The lack of data seriously undermines meaningful, substantial discourse describing data-driven reforms at the federal and institutional level; this problem is particularly acute for students attending HBCUs, TCUs, and community colleges. Researchers pointing to lack of data also identify the culture of the two-year college, which by and large is not set up to support a research friendly culture.

- Collect more longitudinal data that can be disaggregated in terms of
  - Institutional and program types such as community colleges, MSIs, graduate programs, and medical programs
  - Student identities including gender, race and ethnicity, disability, first-generation, nation of origin, documentation, student-athletes, post-traditional and non-traditional students, students with dependents, sexual and gender minorities, and military service and veteran status
  - Previous experiences with mental health, substance use, and trauma
  - Differences in student mental health and substance use issues by discipline and professional field
- Explore models of research partnership between under-resourced institutions, such as community colleges, and researchers at well-resourced institutions that can develop meaningful data for under-resourced institutions
- Develop, support, and maintain an ongoing, longitudinal national monitoring system that identifies student death by suicide
- Conduct systematic evaluation of the outcomes of specific mental health services and programs

References

AACC (American Association of Community Colleges). 2019. *Community college enrollment crisis? Historical trends in community college enrollment.* Washington, DC. https://www.aacc.nche.edu/wp-content/uploads/2019/08/Crisis-in-Enrollment-2019.pdf.

AAMC (Association of American Medical Colleges). 2019. 2019 facts: Enrollment, graduates, and MD/PhD data. Washington, DC.

AAU (Association of American Universities). 2019. AAU campus climate survey (2019). https://www.aau.edu/key-issues/campus-climate-and-safety/aau-campus-climate-survey-2019 (accessed December 9, 2020).

ACCA (American College Counseling Association). 2020. Professional advocacy and public awareness (PAPA) paper: Outsourcing of counseling services. Alexandria, VA.

ACE (American Council on Education). 2020. College and university presidents respond to COVID-19: 2020 fall term survey, part II. Washington, DC.

ACHA. 2012. *American College Health Association-National College Health Assessment II: Undergraduate reference group; Executive summary, spring 2012.* Hanover, MD. https://www.acha.org/documents/ncha/ACHA-NCHA-II_ReferenceGroup_ExecutiveSummary_Spring2012.pdf.

ACHA. 2014. *American College Health Association-National College Health Assessment II: Reference group data report, fall 2013.* Hanover, MD. https://www.acha.org/documents/ncha/ACHA-NCHA-II_ReferenceGroup_DataReport_Fall2013.pdf.

ACHA. 2016. *Addressing sexual and relationship violence on college and university campuses.* Silver Spring, MD: https://www.acha.org/documents/resources/guidelines/Addressing_Sexual_Violence.pdf (accessed January 5, 2021).

ACHA. 2019a. *American College Health Association-National College Health Assessment IIc: Reference group data report, spring 2019.* Hanover, MD. https://www.acha.org/documents/ncha/NCHA-II_SPRING_2019_US_REFERENCE_GROUP_DATA_REPORT.pdf.

ACHA. 2019b. *Outsourcing of college health programs.* Hanover, MD.

Active Minds. 2020. *COVID-19 impact on college student mental health.* Washington, DC.

ADA National Network. 2020. About the ADA National Network. https://adata.org/about-ada-national-network (accessed September 30, 2020).

ADAA. 2020. PsyberGuide. Silver Spring, MD. https://adaa.org/psyberguide (accessed September 24, 2020).

Advokat, C., and M. Scheithauer. 2013. Attention-deficit hyperactivity disorder (ADHD) stimulant medications as cognitive enhancers. *Frontiers in Neuroscience* 7:82.

Ahmad, F., C. El Morr, P. Ritvo, N. Othman, R. Moineddin, and MVC Team. 2020. An eight-week, web-based mindfulness virtual community intervention for students' mental health: Randomized controlled trial. *JMIR Mental Health* 7(2):e15520-e15520. doi: 10.2196/15520.

Ahn, J. 2011. The effect of social network sites on adolescents' social and academic development: Current theories and controversies. *Journal of the American Society for Information Science and Technology* 62(8):1435-1445.

Aikins, R. D., A. Golub, and A. S. Bennett. 2015. Readjustment of urban veterans: A mental health and substance use profile of Iraq and Afghanistan veterans in higher education. *Journal of American College Health* 63(7):482-494.

Albright, G. 2018. *At-risk simulation: Hispanic/Latinx student study.* New York: Kognito.

Albright, G., and J. T. McMillan. 2018. Virtual humans: Transforming mHealth for veterans with post-traumatic stress disorder (PTSD). *mHealth* 4(3). doi: 10.21037/mhealth.2018.03.03.

Alexander, A., and D. Iarovici. 2018. Graduate students and postdoctoral fellows. Pp. 459-470 in *Student mental health: A guide for psychiatrists, psychologists, and leaders serving in higher education,* L. W. Roberts, ed. Washington, DC: American Psychiatric Association.

Alvesson, M., and S. Sveningsson. 2016. *Changing organizational culture: Culture change work in progress.* 2nd ed. Abingdon, UK: Routledge.

American Psychiatric Association. 2018. Warning signs of mental illness. Washington, DC. https://www.psychiatry.org/patients-families/warning-signs-of-mental-illness (accessed April 3, 2020).

American Psychiatric Association. 2020a. Best practices, policy considerations and COVID-19. Washington, DC. https://www.psychiatry.org/File%20Library/Psychiatrists/Practice/Telepsychiatry/APA-College-Mental-Health-Telepsychiatry-COVID-19.pdf (accessed December 9, 2020).

American Psychiatric Association. 2020b. *Psychiatrists' use of telepsychiatry during COVID-19 public health emergency.* Washington, DC. https://www.psychiatry.org/File%20Library/Psychiatrists/Practice/Telepsychiatry/APA-Telehealth-Survey-2020.pdf (accessed November 20, 2020).

American Psychological Association. 2020. Disability Resources Toolbox (DART). Washington, DC. https://www.apa.org/pi/disability/dart (accessed September 30, 2020).

Anders, S. L., P. A. Frazier, and S. L. Shallcross. 2012. Prevalence and effects of life event exposure among undergraduate and community college students. *Journal of Counseling Psychology* 59(3):449-457.

Anderson, G. 2019. Defunding student mental health. Inside Higher Ed, October 18. https://www.insidehighered.com/news/2019/10/18/mental-health-low-priority-community-colleges (accessed September 28, 2020).

Andrews, F. M., and D. B. Withey. 1976. *Social indicators of well-being.* New York: Plenum Press.

Armstrong, T. 2017. Neurodiversity: The future of special education. *Educational Leadership* 74(7):10-16.

Arnekrans, A. K., S. A. Calmes, J. M. Laux, C. P. Roseman, N. J. Piazza, J. L. Reynolds, D. Harmening, and H. L. Scott. 2018. College students' experiences of childhood developmental traumatic stress: Resilience, first-year academic performance, and substance use. *Journal of College Counseling* 21(1):2-14.

Arria, A. M., K. M. Caldeira, K. B. Vincent, E. R. Winick, R. A. Baron, and K. E. O'Grady. 2013. Discontinuous college enrollment: Associations with substance use and mental health. *Psychiatric Services* 64(2):165-172.

Associated Press. 2020. Colleges are getting slammed amid the coronavirus crisis—and the worst may still lie ahead. *Fortune*, April 7.

Auerbach, R. P., P. Mortier, R. Bruffaerts, J. Alonso, C. Benjet, P. Cuijpers, K. Demyttenaere, D. D. Ebert, J. G. Green, P. Hasking, E. Murray, M. K. Nock, S. Pinder-Amaker, N. A. Sampson, D. J. Stein, G. Vilagut, A. M. Zaslavsky, and R. C. Kessler. 2018. WHO World Mental Health Surveys International College Student Project: Prevalence and distribution of mental disorders. *Journal of Abnormal Psychology* 127(7):623-638. doi: 10.1037/abn0000362.

Austin, A., H. Herrick, and S. Proescholdbell. 2015. Adverse childhood experiences related to poor adult health among lesbian, gay, and bisexual individuals. *American Journal of Public Health* 106(2):314-320.

Ayala, E. E., D. Roseman, J. S. Winseman, and H. R. C. Mason. 2017. Prevalence, perceptions, and consequences of substance use in medical students. *Medical Education Online* 22(1):1392824.

Baik, C., W. Larcombe, and A. Brooker. 2019. How universities can enhance student mental wellbeing: The student perspective. *Higher Education Research and Development* 38(4):674-687.

Baker, M. R., P. A. Frazier, C. Greer, J. A. Paulsen, K. Howard, L. N. Meredith, S. L. Anders, and S. L. Shallcross. 2016. Sexual victimization history predicts academic performance in college women. *Journal of Counseling Psychology* 63(6):685-692.

Barker, G., A. Olukoya, and P. Aggleton. 2005. Young people, social support and help-seeking. *International Journal of Adolescent Medicine and Health* 17(4):315-335.

Bartgis, J., and G. Albright. 2016. Online role-play simulations with emotionally responsive avatars for the early detection of Native youth psychological distress, including depression and suicidal ideation. *American Indian and Alaska Native Mental Health Research* 23(2):1-27.

Baselon, D., K. Bower, L. Carty, A. Chappell, E. Coakley, J. Fann, E. Lind, A. Malmon, R. MacKay, W. McLaughlin, A. Pappas, R. Szabo, A. White, and L. Wood. 2008. *Campus mental health: Know your rights!* Washington, DC: Judge David L. Bazelon Center for Mental Health Law.

Bendak, S., A. M. Shikhli, and R. H. Abdel-Razek. 2020. How changing organizational culture can enhance innovation: Development of the innovative culture enhancement framework. *Cogent Business and Management* 7(1):1712125. https://doi.org/10.1080/23311975.2020.1712125.

Berger, T., K. Hämmerli, N. Gubser, G. Andersson, and F. Caspar. 2011. Internet-based treatment of depression: A randomized controlled trial comparing guided with unguided self-help. *Cognitive Behaviour Therapy* 40(4):251-266.

Berger, T., J. Boettcher, and F. Caspar. 2014. Internet-based guided self-help for several anxiety disorders: A randomized controlled trial comparing a tailored with a standardized disorder-specific approach. *Psychotherapy (Chic)* 51(2):207-219.

Bishop, T. F., J. K. Seirup, H. A. Pincus, and J. S. Ross. 2016. Population of U.S. practicing psychiatrists declined, 2003–13, which may help explain poor access to mental health care. *Health Affairs* 35(7):1271-1277.

Bloodgood, R. A., J. G. Short, J. M. Jackson, and J. R. Martindale. 2009. A change to pass/fail grading in the first two years at one medical school results in improved psychological well-being. *Academic Medicine* 84(5):655-662.

Bornheimer, L., and J. Gangwisch. 2009. Sports participation as a protective factor against depression and suicidal ideation in adolescents as mediated by self-esteem and social support. *Journal of Developmental and Behavioral Pediatrics* 30:376-384.

Borsari, B., J. G. Murphy, and N. P. Barnett. 2007. Predictors of alcohol use during the first year of college: Implications for prevention. *Addictive Behaviors* 32(10):2062-2086.

Brandtzaeg, P. B., A. Pultier, and G. M. Moen. 2018. Losing control to data-hungry apps: A mixed-methods approach to mobile app privacy. *Social Science Computer Review* 37(4):466-488.

Breitschuh, V., and J. Göretz. 2019. User motivation and personal safety on a mobile dating app. In *Social computing and social media: Design, human behavior and analytics*, G. Meiselwitz, ed. HCII 2019. Lecture Notes in Computer Science, vol. 11578. Springer, Cham. https://doi.org/10.1007/978-3-030-21902-4_20.

Breslau, J., M. Lane, N. Sampson, and R. C. Kessler. 2008. Mental disorders and subsequent educational attainment in a U.S. national sample. *Journal of Psychiatric Research* 42(9):708-716.

Broglio, S. P., M. McCrea, T. McAllister, J. Harezlak, B. Katz, D. Hack, and B. Hainline. 2017. A national study on the effects of concussion in collegiate athletes and U.S. military service academy members: The NCAA-DoD Concussion Assessment, Research and Education (CARE) Consortium structure and methods. *Sports Medicine* 47(7):1437-1451. doi: 10.1007/s40279-017-0707-1.

Brown, S. 2020. *Overwhelmed: The real campus mental-health crisis and new models for well-being.* Washington, DC: The Chronicle of Higher Education. https://store.chronicle.com/products/overwhelmed (accessed December 26, 2020).

Brownson, C., D. J. Drum, S. E. Smith, and A. Burton Denmark. 2011. Differences in suicidal experiences of male and female undergraduate and graduate students. *Journal of College Student Psychotherapy* 25(4):277-294.

Brownson, C., M. S. Becker, R. Shadick, S. S. Jaggars, and Y. Nitkin-Kaner. 2014. Suicidal behavior and help seeking among diverse college students. *Journal of College Counseling* 17(2):116-130.

Bruce-Sanford, G., and L. Soares. 2019. Mental health and post-traditional learners. *Higher Education Today*, April 22. Washington, DC: American Council on Education.

Brunsma, D. L., D. G. Embrick, and J. H. Shin. 2016. Graduate students of color: Race, racism, and mentoring in the white waters of academia. *Sociology of Race and Ethnicity* 3(1):1-13.

Byrd, D. R., and K. J. McKinney. 2012. Individual, interpersonal, and institutional level factors associated with the mental health of college students. *Journal of American College Health* 60(3):185-193.

Cabral, R. R., and T. B. Smith. 2011. Racial/ethnic matching of clients and therapists in mental health services: A meta-analytic review of preferences, perceptions, and outcomes. *Journal of Counseling Psychology* 58(4):537-554. doi: 10.1037/a0025266.

Cadigan, J. M., and C. M. Lee. 2019. Identifying barriers to mental health service utilization among heavy drinking community college students. *Community College Journal of Research and Practice* 43(8):585-594.

Cain, J. 2018. It's time to confront student mental health issues associated with smartphones and social media. *American Journal of Pharmaceutical Education* 82(7):6862.

CAMHI (Child and Adolescent Health Measurement Initiative). 2018. *Adverse childhood experiences among U.S. children.* Baltimore, MD. https://www.cahmi.org/wp-content/uploads/2018/05/aces_fact_sheet.pdf (January 5, 2021).

Canby, N., I. Cameron, A. Calhoun, and G. Buchanan. 2015. A brief mindfulness intervention for healthy college students and its effects on psychological distress, self-control, meta-mood, and subjective vitality. *Mindfulness* 6.

Capatides, C. 2020. Colleges across the U.S. brace for impact as the coronavirus batters their already tenuous financial ground. CBS News, April 10. https://www.cbsnews.com/news/us-colleges-coronavirus-impact-finances (accessed April 21, 2020).

Carlson, E. J., M. S. Poole, N. J. Lambert, and J. C. Lammers. 2016. A study of organizational responses to dilemmas in interorganizational emergency management. *Communication Research* 44(2):287-315. https://doi.org/10.1177/0093650215621775.

Carter, A. C., K. O. Brandon, and M. S. Goldman. 2010. The college and noncollege experience: A review of the factors that influence drinking behavior in young adulthood. *Journal of Studies on Alcohol and Drugs* 71(5):742-750.

Casseus, M., B. West, J. M. Graber, O. Wackowski, J. M. Cooney, and H. S. Lee. 2020. Disparities in illicit drug use and disability status among a nationally representative sample of U.S. college students. *Disability and Health Journal* 14(1):00949. https://doi.org/10.1016/j.dhjo.2020.100949.

Cauce, A. M. 2019. Using psychology for the public good: Making higher education accessible for low-income students. *Perspectives on Psychological Science* 14(1):70-73.

CBHSQ (Center for Behavioral Health Statistics and Quality). 2019. *Key substance use and mental health indicators in the United States: Results from the 2018 National Survey on Drug Use and Health.* HHS publication no. Pep19-5068, NSDUH Series H-54. Rockville, MD: Substance Abuse and Mental Health Services Administration.

CCMH (Center for Collegiate Mental Health). 2015. *Center for Collegiate Mental Health 2014 annual report.* State College: Pennsylvania State University.

CCMH. 2017. *2016 annual report.* State College: Pennsylvania State University.

CCMH. 2018. *Center for Collegiate Mental Health 2017 annual report.* State College: Pennsylvania State University. Publication no. STA 18-166.

CCMH. 2020a. *Center for Collegiate Mental Health 2019 annual report.* State College: Pennsylvania State University.

CCMH. 2020b. *The clinical load index.* State College: Pennsylvania State University.

CDC (Centers for Disease Control and Prevention). 2018. Well-being concepts. Atlanta, GA. https://www.cdc.gov/hrqol/wellbeing.htm#three (accessed April 3, 2020).

CDC. 2019. Death rates due to suicide and homicide among persons aged 10–24: United States, 2000–2017. Atlanta, GA. https://www.cdc.gov/nchs/products/databriefs/db352.htm (accessed December 9, 2020).

Chapman, E. N., A. Kaatz, and M. Carnes. 2013. Physicians and implicit bias: How doctors may unwittingly perpetuate health care disparities. *Journal of General Internal Medicine* 28(11):1504-1510.

Chen, J. I., G. D. Romero, and M. S. Karver. 2016. The relationship of perceived campus culture to mental health help-seeking intentions. *Journal of Counseling Psychology* 63(6):677-684.

Chen, J. A., C. Stevens, S. H. M. Wong, and C. H. Liu. 2019. Psychiatric symptoms and diagnoses among U.S. college students: A comparison by race and ethnicity. *Psychiatric Services* 70(6):442-449.

Cheng, H. L., K. L. Kwan, and T. Sevig. 2013. Racial and ethnic minority college students' stigma associated with seeking psychological help: Examining psychocultural correlates. *Journal of Counseling Psychology* 60(1):98-111.

Chiauzzi, E., E. Donovan, R. Black, E. Cooney, A. Buechner, and M. Wood. 2011. A survey of 100 community colleges on student substance use, programming, and collaborations. *Journal of American College Health* 59(6):563-573.

Choate, L. H., and S. L. Smith. 2003. Enhancing development in 1st-year college student success courses: A holistic approach. *Journal of Humanistic Counseling, Education and Development* 42(Fall):178-193.

Choi, D., I.-S. Oh, and A. E. Colbert. 2015. Understanding organizational commitment: A meta-analytic examination of the roles of the five-factor model of personality and culture. *Journal of Applied Psychology* 100(5):1542-1567. doi: 10.1037/apl0000014.

Chou, H.-T. G., and N. Edge. 2011. "They are happier and having better lives than I am": The impact of using Facebook on perceptions of others' lives. *Cyberpsychology, Behavior, and Social Networking* 15(2):117-121.

Christens, B. D., and P. T. Inzeo. 2015. Widening the view: Situating collective impact among frameworks for community-led change. *Community Development* 46(4):420-435.

Clance, P. R., and S. A. Imes. 1978. The imposter phenomenon in high-achieving women: Dynamics and therapeutic intervention. *Psychotherapy: Theory, Research and Practice* 15(3):241-247.

Clarke, N., S. Y. Kim, H. R. White, Y. Jiao, and E. Y. Mun. 2013. Associations between alcohol use and alcohol-related negative consequences among Black and white college men and women. *Journal of Studies on Alcohol and Drugs* 74(4):521-531.

CMHC (Counseling and Mental Health Center). 2020. For mental health and medical professionals: State-by-state guide to the rules/laws about telehealth/telemedicine services across state lines. Austin, TX. https://cmhc.utexas.edu/state_telehealth.html (accessed December 15, 2020).

Coduti, W. A., J. A. Hayes, B. D. Locke, and S. J. Youn. 2016. Mental health and professional help-seeking among college students with disabilities. *Rehabilitation Psychology* 61(3):288-296.

Collins, M. E., and C. T. Mowbray. 2005. Higher education and psychiatric disabilities: National survey of campus disability services. *American Journal of Orthopsychiatry* 75(2):304-315.

Conley, C. S., L. V. Travers, and F. B. Bryant. 2013. Promoting psychosocial adjustment and stress management in first-year college students: The benefits of engagement in a psychosocial wellness seminar. *Journal of American College Health* 61(2):75-86.

Cook-Sather, A. 2018. Listening to equity-seeking perspectives: How students' experiences of pedagogical partnership can inform wider discussions of student success. *Higher Education Research and Development* 37(5):923-936.

Cornell University. 2020. CALS peer mentors support new first-generation students. Ithaca, NY. https://news.cornell.edu/stories/2020/09/cals-peer-mentors-support-new-first-generation-students (accessed November 19, 2020).

Cranford, J., D. Eisenberg, and A. Serras. 2009. Substance use behaviors, mental health problems, and use of mental health services in a probability sample of college students. *Addictive Behaviors* 34(2):134-145.

Crenshaw, K. 1989. Demarginalizing the intersection of race and sex: A Black feminist critique of antidiscrimination doctrine, feminist theory and antiracist politics. *University of Chicago Legal Forum* 1989:139-167.

Cropps, T. A., and L. T. Esters. 2018. Sisters, other-mothers, and aunties: The importance of informal mentors for Black women graduate students at predominantly white institutions. *Diverse: Issues in Higher Education*, July 10. https://diverseeducation.com/article/119653/ (accessed September 28, 2020).

Curtin, N., A. J. Stewart, and J. M. Ostrove. 2013. Fostering academic self-concept: Advisor support and sense of belonging among international and domestic graduate students. *American Educational Research Journal* 50(1):108-137.

Curtin, S., and M. Heron. 2019. Death rates due to suicide and homicide among persons aged 10-24: United States, 2000-2017. NCHS Data Brief No. 352 (October):1-8. https://www.cdc.gov/nchs/data/databriefs/db352-h.pdf.

Cuseo, J. B. 1997. *Freshman orientation seminar at community colleges: A research-based rationale for its value, content, and delivery.* ERIC Number ED411005. Arlington, VA: Marymount College. https://eric.ed.gov/?id=ED411005.

Custer, B., and R. Kent. 2019. Understanding the Drug-Free Schools and Communities Act, then and now. *Journal of College and University Law* 44(2):137-159.

Dang, J., K. M. King, and M. Inzlicht. 2020. Why are self-report and behavioral measures weakly correlated? *Trends in Cognitive Sciences* 24(4):267-269.

Danowitz, A., and K. Beddoes. 2018. Characterizing mental health and wellness in students across engineering disciplines. ASEE Conferences, April 29, 2018. https://peer.asee.org/29522 (accessed December 28, 2020).

Davidson, S. 2017. *Trauma-informed practices for postsecondary education: A guide.* Portland, OR: Education Northwest.

Davies, E. B., R. Morriss, and C. Glazebrook. 2014. Computer-delivered and web-based interventions to improve depression, anxiety, and psychological well-being of university students: A systematic review and meta-analysis. *Journal of Medical Internet Research* 16(5):e130.

Dawson, D. A., B. F. Grant, F. S. Stinson, and P. S. Chou. 2004. Another look at heavy episodic drinking and alcohol use disorders among college and noncollege youth. *Journal of Studies on Alcohol and Drugs* 65(4):477-488.

DeLisa, J. A., and J. J. Lindenthal. 2012. Commentary: Reflections on diversity and inclusion in medical education. *Academic Medicine* 87(11):1461-1463.

DeRicco, B. 2006. *Complying with the Drug-Free Schools and Campuses Regulations [EDGAR Part 86]: A guide for university and college administrators.* Washington, DC: Department of Education, Office of Safe and Drug-Free Schools, Higher Education Center for Alcohol and Other Drug Abuse and Violence Prevention.

Diener, E. 2000. Subjective well-being: The science of happiness and a proposal for a national index. *American Psychologist* 55(1):34-43.

DOJ (Department of Justice). 1990. Introduction to the ADA. Washington, DC. https://www.ada.gov/ada_intro.htm#:~:text=To%20be%20protected%20by%20the,as%20having%20such%20an%20impairment (accessed September 24, 2020).

Douce, L. A., and R. P. Keeling. 2014. *A strategic primer on college student mental health.* Washington, DC: American Council on Education.

Duffy, A., K. E. A. Saunders, G. S. Malhi, S. Patten, A. Cipriani, S. H. McNevin, E. MacDonald, and J. Geddes. 2019. Mental health care for university students: A way forward? *Lancet Psychiatry* 6(11):885-887.

Duffy, A., C. Keown-Stoneman, S. Goodday, J. Horrocks, M. Lowe, N. King, W. Pickett, S. H. McNevin, S. Cunningham, D. Rivera, L. Bisdounis, C. R. Bowie, K. Harkness, and K. E. A. Saunders. 2020. Predictors of mental health and academic outcomes in first-year university students: Identifying prevention and early-intervention targets. *BJPsych Open* 6(3):e46.

Duffy, M. E., J. M. Twenge, and T. E. Joiner. 2019. Trends in mood and anxiety symptoms and suicide-related outcomes among U.S. undergraduates, 2007-2018: Evidence from two national surveys. *Journal of Adolescent Health* 65(5):590-598.

Duncan, R. D. 2000. Childhood maltreatment and college drop-out rates: Implications for child abuse researchers. *Journal of Interpersonal Violence* 15(9):987-995.

Dundar, A., and D. Shapiro. 2016. *The National Student Clearinghouse as an integral part of the national postsecondary data infrastructure*. National Student Clearinghouse Research Center. http://www.ihep.com/sites/default/files/uploads/postsecdata/docs/resources/national_student_clearinghouse.pdf.

Dvořáková, K., M. Kishida, J. Li, S. Elavsky, P. C. Broderick, M. R. Agrusti, and M. T. Greenberg. 2017. Promoting healthy transition to college through mindfulness training with first-year college students: Pilot randomized controlled trial. *Journal of American College Health* 65(4):259-267.

Dyrbye, L. N., C. P. West, D. Satele, S. Boone, L. Tan, J. Sloan, and T. D. Shanafelt. 2014. Burnout among U.S. medical students, residents, and early career physicians relative to the general U.S. population. *Academic Medicine* 89(3):443-451.

ED (Department of Education). 2020. Family Educational Rights and Privacy Act of 1974. Washington, DC. https://www.ed.gov/policy/gen/guid/fpco/ferpa/index.html (accessed December 14, 2020).

Edman, J. L., S. B. Watson, and D. J. Patron. 2016. Trauma and psychological distress among ethnically diverse community college students. *Community College Journal of Research and Practice* 40(4):335-342.

Edmondson, A. C., and Z. Lei. 2014. Psychological safety: The history, renaissance, and future of an interpersonal construct. *Annual Review of Organizational Psychology and Organizational Behavior* 1:23-43. https://doi.org/10.1146/annurev-orgpsych-031413-091305.

Edwards, J., and A. Lenhart. 2017. Survey of community/two-year college counseling services, 2016-2017.

Eisenberg, D., E. Golberstein, and S. E. Gollust. 2007. Help-seeking and access to mental health care in a university student population. *Medical Care* 45(7):594-601.

Eisenberg, D., E. Golberstein, and J. Hunt. 2009. Mental health and academic success in college. *B.E. Journal of Economic Analysis and Policy* 9. https://doi.org/10.2202/1935-1682.2191.

Eisenberg, D., J. Hunt, and N. Speer. 2013. Mental health in American colleges and universities: Variation across student subgroups and across campuses. *Journal of Nervous and Mental Disease* 201(1):60-67.

Eisenberg, D., S. Goldrick-Rab, S. K. Lipson, and K. Broton. 2016. *Too distressed to learn? Mental health among community college students*. Madison, WI: Wisconsin HOPE Lab.

Eisenberg, D., S. K. Lipson, P. Ceglarek, M. Phillips, S. Zhou, J. Morigney, A. Talaski, and S. Steverson. 2019. *The Healthy Minds Study: 2018-2019 data report*. Ann Arbor: University of Michigan.

Ellis, D. 2017. *Becoming a master student*. 17th ed. Independence, KY: Cengage Learning.

Espinosa, L. L., J. Turk, and M. Taylor. 2018. *Pulling back the curtain: Enrollment and outcomes at minority serving institutions*. Washington, DC: American Council on Education Center for Policy Research and Strategy. https://www.acenet.edu/Documents/Pulling-Back-the-Curtain-Enrollment-and-Outcomes-at-MSIs.pdf (accessed September 30, 2020).

Espinosa, L. L., J. M. Turk, M. Taylor, and H. M. Chessman. 2019. *Race and ethnicity in higher education: A status report.* Washington, DC: American Council on Higher Education.

Evans, T. M., L. Bira, J. B. Gastelum, L. T. Weiss, and N. L. Vanderford. 2018. Evidence for a mental health crisis in graduate education. *Nature Biotechnology* 36(3):282-284.

Feldblum, M., S. Hubbard, A. Lim, C. Penichet-Paul, and H. Siegel. 2020. *Undocumented students in higher education.* Washington, DC: Presidents' Alliance on Higher Education and Immigration.

Felitti, V. J., R. F. Anda, D. Nordenberg, D. F. Williamson, A. M. Spitz, V. Edwards, M. P. Koss, and J. S. Marks. 1998. Relationship of childhood abuse and household dysfunction to many of the leading causes of death in adults. The Adverse Childhood Experiences (ACE) Study. *American Journal of Preventive Medicine* 14(4):245-258.

Figueiredo, A. R., and T. Abreu. 2015. Suicide among LGBT individuals. *European Psychiatry* 30:1815.

García, I. O., and S. J. Henderson. 2014. Mentoring experiences of Latina graduate students. *Multicultural Learning and Teaching* 10(1):91-110.

Gary, F. A. 2005. Stigma: Barrier to mental health care among ethnic minorities. *Issues in Mental Health Nursing* 26(10):979-999.

Gibbons, R. D., and F. V. deGruy. 2019. Without wasting a word: Extreme improvements in efficiency and accuracy using computerized adaptive testing for mental health disorders (CAT-MH). *Current Psychiatry Reports* 21(8):67.

Gibbons, R. D., and D. R. Hedeker. 1992. Full-information item bi-factor analysis. *Psychometrika* 57(3):423-436.

Gibbons, R. D., R. D. Bock, D. Hedeker, D. J. Weiss, E. Segawa, D. K. Bhaumik, D. J. Kupfer, E. Frank, V. J. Grochocinski, and A. Stover. 2007. Full-information item bi-factor analysis of graded response data. *Applied Psychological Measurement* 31(1):4-19.

Gobbi, G., T. Atkin, T. Zytynski, S. Wang, S. Askari, J. Boruff, M. Ware, N. Marmorstein, A. Cipriani, N. Dendukuri, and N. Mayo. 2019. Association of cannabis use in adolescence and risk of depression, anxiety, and suicidality in young adulthood: A systematic review and meta-analysis. *JAMA Psychiatry* 76(4):426-434.

Godoy Garraza, L., S. Peart Boyce, C. Walrath, D. B. Goldston, and R. McKeon. 2018. An economic evaluation of the Garrett Lee Smith Memorial Suicide Prevention Program. *Suicide and Life-Threatening Behavior* 48(1):3-11.

Graham, I. D., J. Logan, M. B. Harrison, S. E. Straus, J. Tetroe, W. Caswell, and N. Robinson. 2006. Lost in knowledge translation: Time for a map? *Journal of Continuing Education in the Health Professions* 26(1):13-24.

Green, A. 2019. *Emotion and cognition in the age of AI.* London, UK: Economist Intelligence Unit.

Green, A. R., D. R. Carney, D. J. Pallin, L. H. Ngo, K. L. Raymond, L. I. Iezzoni, and M. R. Banaji. 2007. Implicit bias among physicians and its prediction of thrombolysis decisions for Black and white patients. *Journal of General Internal Medicine* 22(9):1231-1238.

Guille, C., H. Speller, R. Laff, C. N. Epperson, and S. Sen. 2010. Utilization and barriers to mental health services among depressed medical interns: A prospective multisite study. *Journal of Graduate Medical Education* 2(2):210-214.

Hadlaczky, G., S. Hökby, A. Mkrtchian, V. Carli, and D. Wasserman. 2014. Mental health first aid is an effective public health intervention for improving knowledge, attitudes, and behaviour: A meta-analysis. *International Review of Psychiatry* 26(4):467-475.

Haidt, J., and J. M. Twenge. 2019. Is there an increase in adolescent mood disorders, self-harm, and suicide since 2010 in the USA and UK? A review. https://docs.google.com/document/d/1diMvsMeRphUH7E6D1d_J7R6WbDdgnzFHDHPx9HXzR5o/edit (accessed November 19, 2020).

Ham, L. S., and D. A. Hope. 2003. College students and problematic drinking: A review of the literature. *Clinical Psychology Review* 23(5):719-759.

Hardner, K., M. R. Wolf, and E. S. Rinfrette. 2018. Examining the relationship between higher educational attainment, trauma symptoms, and internalizing behaviors in child sexual abuse survivors. *Child Abuse and Neglect* 86:375-383.

Harrer, M., S. H. Adam, H. Baumeister, P. Cuijpers, E. Karyotaki, R. P. Auerbach, R. C. Kessler, R. Bruffaerts, M. Berking, and D. D. Ebert. 2019. Internet interventions for mental health in university students: A systematic review and meta-analysis. *International Journal of Methods in Psychiatric Research* 28(2):e1759.

Harrison-Bernard, L. M., A. C. Augustus-Wallace, F. M. Souza-Smith, F. Tsien, G. P. Casey, and T. P. Gunaldo. 2020. Knowledge gains in a professional development workshop on diversity, equity, inclusion, and implicit bias in academia. *Advances in Physiology Education* 44(3):286-294.

Hartley, M. T. 2011. Examining the relationships between resilience, mental health, and academic persistence in undergraduate college students. *Journal of American College Health* 59(7):596-604.

Hayes, J. A., S. J. Youn, L. G. Castonguay, B. D. Locke, A. A. McAleavey, and S. Nordberg. 2011. Rates and predictors of counseling center use among college students of color. *Journal of College Counseling* 14(2):105–116.

Hayes, J. A., J. Petrovich, R. A. Janis, Y. Yang, L. G. Castonguay, and B. D. Locke. 2020. Suicide among college students in psychotherapy: Individual predictors and latent classes. *Journal of Counseling Psychology* 67(1):104-114.

Hazelrigg, K., and M. Woodworth. 2019. *New initiative to support graduate student mental health and wellness.* Washington, DC: Council of Graduate Schools.

HBFF (Hazelden Betty Ford Foundation). 2017. Collegiate recovery programs gaining strength. Emerging Drug Trends, September. Center City, MN. https://www.hazeldenbettyford.org/education/bcr/addiction-research/collegiate-recovery-edt-917 (accessed September 30, 2020).

HECADMPR (Higher Education Center for Alcohol and Drug Misuse Prevention and Recovery). 2020. Recovery. Columbus, OH: The Ohio State University. https://hecaod.osu.edu/campus-professionals/recovery-2/.

Hedegaard, Curtin, and Warner, 2020. https://www.cdc.gov/nchs/data/databriefs/db362-h.pdf.

HEMHA (Higher Education Mental Health Alliance). 2012. *Balancing safety and support on campus: A guide for campus teams.* New York.

HEMHA. 2014. *College counseling from a distance: Deciding whether and when to engage in telemental health services.* New York.

HEMHA. 2019. *HEMHA guide: College counseling from a distance: Deciding whether and when to engage in telemental health services.* New York. http://hemha.org/wp-content/uploads/2019/01/HEMHA-Distance-Counseling_FINAL2019.pdf (accessed September 30, 2020).

HHS and ED (Department of Health and Human Services and Department of Education). 2019. *Joint guidance on the application of the Family Educational Rights and Privacy Act (FERPA) and the Health Insurance Portability and Acountability Act of 1996 (HIPAA) to student health records.* Washington, DC: Department of Health and Human Services.

Hingson, R. W., W. Zha, and E. R. Weitzman. 2009. Magnitude of and trends in alcohol-related mortality and morbidity among U.S. college students ages 18-24, 1998-2005. *Journal of Studies on Alcohol and Drugs* 16:12-20.

Hinojosa, R., J. Nguyen, K. Sellers, and H. Elassar. 2019. Barriers to college success among students that experienced adverse childhood events. *Journal of American College Health* 67(6):531-540.

HMN (Healthy Minds Nework). 2013. *Return on investment calculator (R.O.I.) for college mental health services and programs.* Ann Arbor, MI. https://umich.qualtrics.com/jfe/form/SV_6xN9QUSlFtgtRQh (accessed December 9, 2020).

HMN. 2020. Datasets from 2007 through 2019. Ann Arbor, MI. https://healthymindsnetwork.org/research/data-for-researchers/ (accessed accessed January 5, 2020).

HMN and ACHA (Healthy Minds Network and American College Health Association). 2020. *The impact of COVID-19 on college student well-being.* Ann Arbor, MI: Healthy Minds Network.

Howlett, J., and M. Stein. 2016. Post-traumatic stress disorder: Relationship to traumatic brain injury and approach to treatment. In *Translational Research in Traumatic Brain Injury*, G. Grant and D. Laskowitz, eds. Boca Raton, FL: CRC Press/Taylor and Francis Group.

HRCF (Human Rights Campaign Foundation). 2018. *Gender-expansive youth report.* Washington, DC. https://www.hrc.org/resources/2018-gender-expansive-youth-report (accessed December 28, 2020).

HRSA (Health Resources and Services Administration). 2016. *National projections of supply and demand for behavioral health practitioners: 2013-2025.* Rockville, MD: Substance Abuse and Mental Health Services Administration.

Huang, G. C., J. B. Unger, D. Soto, K. Fujimoto, M. A. Pentz, M. Jordan-Marsh, and T. W. Valente. 2014. Peer influences: The impact of online and offline friendship networks on adolescent smoking and alcohol use. *Journal of Adolescent Health* 54(5):508-514.

Huckins, J. F., A. W. daSilva, W. Wang, E. Hedlund, C. Rogers, S. K. Nepal, J. Wu, M. Obuchi, E. I. Murphy, M. L. Meyer, D. D. Wagner, P. E. Holtzheimer, and A. T. Campbell. 2020. Mental health and behavior of college students during the early phases of the COVID-19 pandemic: Longitudinal smartphone and ecological momentary assessment study. *Journal of Medical Internet Research* 22(6):e20185.

IACS (International Accreditation of Counseling Services). 2019. Statement regarding recommended staff to student ratios. Alexandria, VA. https://iacsinc.org/staff-to-student-ratios/ (accessed April 27, 2020).

Iarovici, D. 2014. *Mental health issues and the university student.* Baltimore, MD: Johns Hopkins University Press.

Iarovici, D., and A. Alexander. 2018. Medical students, residents, and fellows. Pp. 471-481 in *Student mental health: A guide for psychiatrists, psychologists, and leaders serving in higher education,* L. W. Roberts, ed. Washington, DC: American Psychiatric Association.

Ingram, L., and B. Wallace. 2018. "It creates fear and divides us": Minority college students' experiences of stress from racism, coping responses, and recommendations for colleges. *Journal of Health Disparities Research and Practice* 12(1), Article 6.

IOM (Institute of Medicine). 2003. *Unequal treatment: Confronting racial and ethnic disparities in health care.* B. D. Smedley, A. Y. Stith, and A. R. Nelson, eds. Washington, DC: The National Academies Press.

IOM. 2015. *Psychosocial interventions for mental and substance use disorders: A framework for establishing evidence-based standards.* M. J. England, A. S. Butler, and M. L. Gonzalez, eds. Washington, DC: The National Academies Press.

Ireland, D. T., K. E. Freeman, C. E. Winston-Proctor, K. D. DeLaine, S. McDonald Lowe, and K. M. Woodson. 2018. (Un)hidden figures: A synthesis of research examining the intersectional experiences of Black women and girls in STEM education. *Review of Research in Education* 42(1):226-254.

Jack, A. A. 2019. *The privileged poor: How elite colleges are failing disadvantaged students.* Cambridge, MA: Harvard University Press.

Jed Foundation. 2016. The Value of Campus Behavioral Intervention Teams. jedfoundation.org/colleges-should-have-behavioral-intervention-teams/ (accessed January 19, 2021).

Jed Foundation. 2008. *Student mental health and the law: A resource for institutions of higher education.* New York.

Jed Foundation. 2013. *Balancing safety and support on campus: A guide for campus teams.* New York: Higher Education Mental Health Alliance. https://www.jedfoundation.org/wp-content/uploads/2016/06/campus_teams_guide.pdf (accessed December 28, 2020).

Jed Foundation and Clinton Foundation. 2014. Help a friend in need. Menlo Park, CA: Facebook.

Jed Foundation and EDC (Education Development Center). 2011. *Guide to campus mental health action planning.* Waltham, MA: Education Development Center.

Johns, M. M., R. Lowry, J. Andrzejewski, L. C. Barrios, Z. Demissie, T. McManus, C. N. Rasberry, L. Robin, and J. M. Underwood. 2019. Transgender identity and experiences of violence victimization, substance use, suicide risk, and sexual risk behaviors among high school students: 19 states and large urban school districts, 2017. *Morbidity and Mortality Weekly Report* 68(3):67-71.

Jones, N., K. Bower, and A. Furuzawa. 2016a. *Back to school: Toolkits to support the full inclusion of students with early psychosis in higher education. Campus staff and administrator version.* Alexandria, VA: National Association of State Mental Health Program Directors.

Jones, N., K. Bower, and A. Furuzawa. 2016b. *Back to school: Toolkits to support the full inclusion of students with early psychosis in higher education. Student and family version.* Alexandria, VA: National Association of State Mental Health Program Directors.

Jorm, A. F., B. A. Kitchener, and N. J. Reavley. 2019. Mental health first aid training: Lessons learned from the global spread of a community education program. *World Psychiatry* 18(2):142-143.

JTFDTGP (Joint Task Force for the Development of Telepsychology Guidelines for Psychologists). 2013. *Guidelines for the practice of telepsychology.* Washington, DC: American Psychological Association.

Jury, M., A. Smeding, N. M. Stephens, J. E. Nelson, C. Aelenei, and C. Darnon. 2017. The experience of low-SES students in higher education: Psychological barriers to success and interventions to reduce social-class inequality. *Journal of Social Issues* 73(1):23-41.

Kafka, A. C. 2019. Overburdened mental-health counselors look after students. But who looks after the counselors? *The Chronicle of Higher Education*, September 18. https://www.chronicle.com/article/overburdened-mental-health-counselors-look-after-students-but-who-looks-after-the-counselors/ (accessed December 15, 2020).

Kalkbrenner, M. T., and K. L. Carlisle. 2019. Faculty members and college counseling: Utility of the REDFLAGS model. *Journal of College Student Psychotherapy.* doi: 10.1080/87568225.2019.1621230.

Kalkbrenner, M. T., C. A. Sink, and J. L. Smith. 2020. Mental health literacy and peer-to-peer counseling referrals among community college students. *Journal of Counseling and Development* 98(2):172-182.

Kalkbrenner, M. T., E. M. Brown, K. L. Carlisle, and R. M. Carlisle. 2019. Utility of the REDFLAGS model for supporting community college students' mental health: Implications for counselors. *Journal of Counseling and Development* 97(4):417-426.

Katz, D. S., and K. Davison. 2014. Community college student mental health:A comparative analysis. *Community College Review* 42(4):307-326.

Kern, A., W. Heininger, E. Klueh, S. Salazar, B. Hansen, T. Meyer, and D. Eisenberg. 2016. Athletes connected: Results from a pilot project to address knowledge and attitudes about mental health among college student-athletes. *Journal of Clinical Sport Psychology* 11(4):324-336.

Kern, A., V. Hong, J. Song, S. K. Lipson, and D. Eisenberg. 2018. Mental health apps in a college setting: Openness, usage, and attitudes. *mHealth* 4(6).

Khan, C. T., and I. Hansen. 2018. Transgender students. Pp. 425-438 in *Student mental health: A guide for psychiatrists, psychologists, and leaders serving in higher education*, L. W. Roberts, ed. Washington, DC: American Psychiatric Association.

King, S. C., Richner, K. A., Tuliao, A. P., Kennedy, J. L., and McChargue, D. E. 2019. A comparison between telehealth and face-to-face delivery of a brief alcohol intervention for college students. *Substance Abuse* 41(4):501–509.

King Lyn, M. M. 2015. Essential services in college counseling. Pp. 41-64 in *The college and university counseling manual*, S. Hodges, K. Shelton, and M. M. King Lyn, eds. New York: Springer Publishing Company.

Kirby, J. B., S. H. Zuvekas, A. E. Borsky, and Q. Ngo-Metzger. 2019. Rural residents with mental health needs have fewer care visits than urban counterparts. *Health Affairs* 38(12):2057-2060.

Kirzinger, A., A. Kearney, L. Hamel, and M. Brodie. 2020. *KFF health tracking poll; Early April 2020; The impact of coronavirus on life in America.* Washington, DC: Kaiser Family Foundation. https://www.kff.org/health-reform/report/kff-health-tracking-poll-early-april-2020/ (accessed April 3, 2020).

Kitchener, B. A., A. F. Jorm, and C. M. Kelly. 2017. *Mental first aid manual.* 4th ed. Melbourne: Mental First Aid Australia.

Kognito. 2016. California community colleges implement Kognito's mental health and suicide prevention simulations to reduce stigma and engage faculty, staff, and students in supporting those who exhibit signs of distress. New York: Kognito.

Kraepelien, M., C. Svanborg, L. Lallerstedt, V. Sennerstam, N. Lindefors, and V. Kaldo. 2019. Individually tailored internet treatment in routine care: A feasibility study. *Internet Interventions* 18:100263.

Kraft, D. P. 2011. One hundred years of college mental health. *Journal of American College Health* 59(6):477-481.

Kuhn, E., and S. McCaslin. 2018. Military and veteran students. Pp. 449-458 in *Student mental health: A guide for psychiatrists, psychologists, and leaders serving in higher education*, L. W. Roberts, ed. Washington, DC: American Psychiatric Association.

Lane, T. 2016. Discrimination in the laboratory: A meta-analysis of economics experiments. *European Economic Review* 90(C):375-402.

Larcombe, W., S. Finch, R. Sore, C. M. Murray, S. Kentish, R. A. Mulder, P. Lee-Stecum, C. Baik, O. Tokatlidis, and D. A. Williams. 2016. Prevalence and socio-demographic correlates of psychological distress among students at an Australian university. *Studies in Higher Education* 41(6):1074-1091.

Lattie, E. G., S. K. Lipson, and D. Eisenberg. 2019. Technology and college student mental health: Challenges and opportunities. *Frontiers in Psychiatry* 10:246.

Lauff, E., X. Chen, and T. Morgan. 2018. *Military service and educational attainment of high school sophomores after 9/11: Experiences of 2002 high school sophomores as of 2012*. NCES 2019-427. Washington, DC: Department of Education. https://nces.ed.gov/pubs2019/2019427.pdf.

Lee, D., E. A. Olson, B. Locke, S. T. Michelson, and E. Odes. 2009. The effects of college counseling services on academic performance and retention. *Journal of College Student Development* 50(3):305-319.

Lee, P. 2011. The curious life of in loco parentis in American universities. *Higher Education in Review* 8:65-90.

Lehmann, J. P., T. G. Davies, and K. M. Laurin. 2000. Listening to student voices about postsecondary education. *Teaching Exceptional Children* 32(5):60-65.

Levecque, K., F. Anseel, A. Beuckelaer, J. Van der Heyden, and L. Gisle. 2017. Work organization and mental health problems in PhD students. *Research Policy* 46(4):868-879.

LeViness, P., C. Bershad, K. Gorman, L. Braun, and T. Murray. 2018. *The Association for University and College Counseling Center Directors annual survey: Public version 2018*. Indianapolis, IN: Association for University and College Counseling Center Directors.

LeViness, P., K. Gorman, L. Braun, L. Koenig, and C. Bershad. 2019. *The Association for University and College Counseling Center Directors Annual Survey: 2019*. Indianapolis, IN: Association for University and College Counseling Center Directors.

Levis, B., A. Benedetti, J. P. A. Ioannidis, Y. Sun, Z. Negeri, C. He, Y. Wu, A. Krishnan, P. M. Bhandari, D. Neupane, M. Imran, D. B. Rice, K. E. Riehm, N. Saadat, M. Azar, J. Boruff, P. Cuijpers, S. Gilbody, L. A. Kloda, D. McMillan, S. B. Patten, I. Shrier, R. C. Ziegelstein, S. H. Alamri, D. Amtmann, L. Ayalon, H. R. Baradaran, A. Beraldi, C. N. Bernstein, A. Bhana, C. H. Bombardier, G. Carter, M. H. Chagas, D. Chibanda, K. Clover, Y. Conwell, C. Diez-Quevedo, J. R. Fann, F. H. Fischer, L. Gholizadeh, L. J. Gibson, E. P. Green, C. G. Greeno, B. J. Hall, E. E. Haroz, K. Ismail, N. Jetté, M. E. Khamseh, Y. Kwan, M. A. Lara, S. I. Liu, S. R. Loureiro, B. Löwe, R. A. Marrie, L. Marsh, A. McGuire, K. Muramatsu, L. Navarrete, F. L. Osório, I. Petersen, A. Picardi, S. L. Pugh, T. J. Quinn, A. G. Rooney, E. H. Shinn, A. Sidebottom, L. Spangenberg, P. L. L. Tan, M. Taylor-Rowan, A. Turner, H. C. van Weert, P. A. Vöhringer, L. I. Wagner, J. White, K. Winkley, and B. D. Thombs. 2020. Patient health questionnaire-9 scores do not accurately estimate depression prevalence: Individual participant data meta-analysis. *Journal of Clinical Epidemiology* 122:115-128.e111.

Lillis, M. P. 2011. Faculty emotional intelligence and student-faculty interactions: Implications for student retention. *Journal of College Student Retention: Research, Theory and Practice* 13(2):155-178.

Lipson, S. K., and N. Roy. 2015. Data-driven approaches to evaluation and improvement of campus mental health services and systems. PowerPoint presentation given in the HMN Webinar Series, session 14, November 2015. https://healthymindsnetwork.org/wp-content/uploads/2019/04/HMN-Webinar-14-11.16.2015.pptx (accessed December 15, 2020).

Lipson, S. K., S. Zhou, B. Wagner, K. Beck, and D. Eisenberg. 2016. Major differences: Variations in undergraduate and graduate student mental health and treatment utilization across academic disciplines. *Journal of College Student Psychotherapy* 30(1):23-41.

Lipson, S. K., A. Kern, D. Eisenberg, and A. M. Breland-Noble. 2018. Mental health disparities among college students of color. *Journal of Adolescent Health* 63(3):348-356.

Lipson, S. K., E. G. Lattie, and D. Eisenberg. 2019. Increased rates of mental health service utilization by U.S. college students: 10-year population-level trends (2007–2017). *Psychiatric Services* 70(1):60-63.

Lipson, S. K., S. Abelson, P. Ceglarek, M. Phillips, and D. Eisenberg. 2019. *Investing in student mental health: Opportunities and benefits for college leadership.* Washington, DC: American Council on Education.

Liu, C. H., C. Stevens, S. H. M. Wong, M. Yasui, and J. A. Chen. 2019. The prevalence and predictors of mental health diagnoses and suicide among U.S. college students: Implications for addressing disparities in service use. *Depression and Anxiety* 36(1):8-17.

Locke, B., J. Buzolits, P.-W. Lei, J. Boswell, A. McAleavey, T. Sevig, J. Dowis, and J. Hayes. 2010. Development of the Counseling Center Assessment of Psychological Symptoms-62 (CCAPS-62). *Journal of Counseling Psychology* 58:97-109.

Lockwood, P., and R. Wohl. 2012. The impact of a 15-week lifetime wellness course on behavior change and self-efficacy in college students. *College Student Journal* 46(3):628-641.

Marconi, A., M. Di Forti, C. M. Lewis, R. M. Murray, and E. Vassos. 2016. Meta-analysis of the association between the level of cannabis use and risk of psychosis. *Schizophrenia Bulletin* 42(5):1262-1269.

Marshall, A. 2016. Suicide prevention interventions for sexual and gender minority youth: An unmet need. *Yale Journal of Biology and Medicine* 89(2):205-213.

Martens, M. P., K. Dams-O'Connor, and N. C. Beck. 2006. A systematic review of college student-athlete drinking: Prevalence rates, sport-related factors, and interventions. *Journal of Substance Abuse Treatment* 31(3):305-316.

Martinez, W., G. B. Hickson, B. M. Miller, D. J. Doukas, J. D. Buckley, J. Song, N. L. Sehgal, J. Deitz, C. H. Braddock, and L. S. Lehmann. 2014. Role-modeling and medical error disclosure: A national survey of trainees. *Academic Medicine* 89(3):482-489.

Masataka, N. 2018. Neurodiversity and artistic performance characteristic of children with autism spectrum disorder. *Frontiers in Psychology* 9:2594.

McAleavey, A. A., S. S. Nordberg, J. A. Hayes, L. G. Castonguay, B. D. Locke, and A. J. Lockard. 2012. Clinical validity of the Counseling Center Assessment of Psychological Symptoms-62 (CCAPS-62): Further evaluation and clinical applications. *Journal of Counseling Psychology* 59(4):575-590.

McAleavey, A. A., S. J. Youn, H. Xiao, L. G. Castonguay, J. A. Hayes, and B. D. Locke. 2017. Effectiveness of routine psychotherapy: Method matters. *Psychotherapy Research* 29(2):139-156. doi: 10.1080/10503307.2017.1395921.

McBride, P. E. 2019. Addressing the lack of mental health services for at-risk students at a two-year community college: A contemporary review. *Community College Journal of Research and Practice* 43(2):146-148.

McCabe, P., and S. Fitzgerald. 2019. Moody's annual higher education survey shows net tuition revenue growth dropping for public and private universities. New York: Moody's Investors Service.

McCabe, S. E., J. R. Knight, C. J. Teter, and H. Wechsler. 2005a. Non-medical use of prescription stimulants among us college students: Prevalence and correlates from a national survey. *Addiction* 100(1):96-106.

McCabe, S. E., C. J. Teter, C. J. Boyd, J. R. Knight, and H. Wechsler. 2005b. Nonmedical use of prescription opioids among U.S. college students: Prevalence and correlates from a national survey. *Addictive Behaviors* 30(4):789-805.

McCall, L. 2005. The complexity of intersectionality. *Signs: Journal of Women in Culture and Society* 30(3):1771-1800.

McLaughlin, C. G. 2004. Delays in treatment for mental disorders and health insurance coverage. *Health Services Research* 39(2):221-224.

MCRCDRP (Maryland Collaborative to Reduce College Drinking and Related Problems). 2013. *Reducing alcohol use and related problems among college students: A guide to best practices.* College Park, MD: Center on Alcohol Marketing and Youth, Johns Hopkins University Bloomberg School of Public Health, Center on Young Adult Health and Development, University of Maryland School of Public Health.

McSwain, C., and A. Cunningham. 2006. *Championing success: A report on the progress of tribal college and university alumni.* Prepared by the Institute for Higher Education Policy. Denver, CO: American Indian College Fund. https://files.eric.ed.gov/fulltext/ED539699.pdf.

Mellins, C. A., K. Walsh, A. L. Sarvet, M. Wall, L. Gilbert, J. S. Santelli, M. Thompson, P. A. Wilson, S. Khan, S. Benson, K. Bah, K. A. Kaufman, L. Reardon, and J. S. Hirsch. 2017. Sexual assault incidents among college undergraduates: Prevalence and factors associated with risk. *PLoS One* 12(11):e0186471.

Metcalfe, S. E., and J. Neubrander. 2016. Social determinants and educational barriers to successful admission to nursing programs for minority and rural students. *Journal of Professional Nursing* 32(5):377-382.

Metzler, M., M. T. Merrick, J. Klevens, K. A. Ports, and D. C. Ford. 2017. Adverse childhood experiences and life opportunities: Shifting the narrative. *Children and Youth Services Review* 72:141-149.

MHA (Mental Health America). 2020a. Mental health and COVID-19: Information and resources. Alexandria, VA. https://mhanational.org/covid19 (accessed May 27, 2020).

MHA. 2020b. The state of mental health in America. Alexandria, VA. https://mhanational.org/issues/state-mental-health-america (accessed December 14, 2020).

Mojtabai, R., E. A. Stuart, I. Hwang, W. W. Eaton, N. Sampson, and R. C. Kessler. 2015. Long-term effects of mental disorders on educational attainment in the national comorbidity survey ten-year follow-up. *Social Psychiatry and Psychiatric Epidemiology* 50(10):1577-1591.

Montgomery, B. L. 2018. Building and sustaining diverse functioning networks using social media and digital platforms to improve diversity and inclusivity. *Frontiers in Digital Humanities* 5(22). https://doi.org/10.3389/fdigh.2018.00022.

Murray, R. M., H. Quigley, D. Quattrone, A. Englund, and M. Di Forti. 2016. Traditional marijuana, high-potency cannabis and synthetic cannabinoids: Increasing risk for psychosis. *World Psychiatry* 15(3):195-204.

NAMI (National Alliance on Mental Illness). 2020. Self-harm. Arlington, VA. https://www.nami.org/About-Mental-Illness/Common-with-Mental-Illness/Self-harm (accessed September 30, 2020).

NASEM (National Academies of Sciences, Engineering, and Medicine). 2016. *Ending discrimination against people with mental and substance use disorders: The evidence for stigma change.* Washington, DC: The National Academies Press.

NASEM 2017.

NASEM. 2018a. *Graduate STEM education for the 21st century.* A. Leshner and L. Scherer, eds. Washington, DC: The National Academies Press.

NASEM. 2018b. *Sexual harassment of women: Climate, culture, and consequences in academic sciences, engineering, and medicine.* P. A. Johnson, S. E. Widnall, and F. F. Benya, eds. Washington, DC: The National Academies Press.

NASEM. 2019a. *Minority Serving Institutions: America's underutilized resource for strengthening the STEM workforce.* L. L. Espinosa, K. McGuire, and L. M. Jackson, eds. Washington, DC: The National Academies Press.

NASEM. 2019b. *The science of effective mentorship in STEMM*. A. Byars-Winston and M. L. Dahlberg, eds. Washington, DC: The National Academies Press.

NASEM. 2019c. *Taking action against clinician burnout: A systems approach to professional well-being*. Washington, DC: The National Academies Press.

NASEM. 2020. *Promoting positive adolescent health behaviors and outcomes: Thriving in the 21st century*. R. Graham and N. F. Kahn, eds. Washington, DC: The National Academies Press.

Naslund, J. A., K. A. Aschbrenner, L. A. Marsch, and S. J. Bartels. 2016. The future of mental health care: Peer-to-peer support and social media. *Epidemiology and Psychiatric Sciences* 25(2):113-122.

NCAA (National Collegiate Athletic Association). 2020. Student-athletes. Indianapolis, IN. http://www.ncaa.org/student-athletes (accessed September 24, 2020).

NCD (National Council on Disability). 2017a. *Mental health on college campuses: Investments, accommodations needed to address student needs*. Washington, DC. https://ncd.gov/sites/default/files/NCD_Mental_Health_Report_508_0.pdf (accessed November 19, 2020).

NCD. 2017b. *National disability policy: A progress report*. Washington, DC. https://ncd.gov/sites/default/files/NCD_A%20Progress%20Report_508.pdf (accessed November 19, 2020).

NCDJ (National Center on Disability and Journalism). 2018. *NCDJ style guide*. Tempe, AZ: Arizona State University.

NCES (National Center for Education Statistics). 1999. *Digest of education statistics 1998*. Washington, DC.

NCES. 2017. *Total fall enrollment in degree-granting postsecondary institutions, by control and classification of institution, level of enrollment, and race/ethnicity of student: 2017*. Washington, DC. https://nces.ed.gov/programs/digest/d18/tables/dt18_306.50.asp (accessed December 15, 2020).

NCES. 2020. Undergraduate enrollment. Washington, DC. https://nces.ed.gov/programs/coe/indicator_cha.asp (accessed December 15, 2020).

Nesheim, B. E., M. J. Guentzel, A. H. Hellogg, W. M. McDonald, C. A. Wells, and E. J. Whitt. 2007. Outcomes for students of student affairs-academic affairs partnership programs. *Journal of College Student Development* 48(4):435-454.

Newton, J., M. Dooris, and J. Wills. 2016. Healthy universities: An example of a whole-system health-promoting setting. *Global Health Promotion* 23(1_suppl):57-65. doi: 10.1177/1757975915601037.

NIAAA (National Institute on Alcohol Abuse and Alcoholism). 2019. *Planning alcohol interventions using NIAAA's College AIM*. Bethesda, MD.

NIDA (National Institute on Drug Abuse). 2020a. *Common comorbidities with substance use disorders research report, part 1: The connection between substance use disorders and mental illness*. Rockville, MD. https://www.drugabuse.gov/publications/research-reports/common-comorbidities-substance-use-disorders/part-1-connection-between-substance-use-disorders-mental-illness (accessed September 30, 2020).

NIDA. 2020b. Commonly used terms in addiction science. Rockville, MD. https://www.drugabuse.gov/publications/media-guide/glossary (accessed January 5, 2021).

NIDA. 2020c. Comorbidity: Substance use disorders and other mental illnesses. Rockville, MD. https://www.drugabuse.gov/publications/drugfacts/comorbidity-substance-use-disorders-other-mental-illnesses (accessed September 30, 2020).

NIDA. 2020d. COVID-19: Potential implications for individuals with substance use disorders. Nora's blog, April 6. Rockville, MD. https://www.drugabuse.gov/about-nida/noras-blog/2020/04/covid-19-potential-implications-individuals-substance-use-disorders (accessed May 27, 2020).

NIMH (National Institute of Mental Health). 2020a. Anxiety disorders. Bethesda, MD. https://www.nimh.nih.gov/health/topics/anxiety-disorders/index.shtml (accessed September 30, 2020).

NIMH. 2020b. Attention-deficit/hyperactivity disorder (ADHD): The basics. Bethesda, MD. https://www.nimh.nih.gov/health/publications/attention-deficit-hyperactivity-disorder-adhd-the-basics/index.shtml (accessed September 30, 2020).

NIMH. 2020c. Autism spectrum disorders (ASD). Bethesda, MD. https://www.nimh.nih.gov/health/trials/autism-spectrum-disorders-asd.shtml (accessed September 30, 2020).

NIMH. 2020d. Bipolar disorder. Bethesda, MD. https://www.nimh.nih.gov/health/topics/bipolar-disorder/index.shtml (accessed September 30, 2020).

NIMH. 2020e. Depression. Bethesda, MD. https://www.nimh.nih.gov/health/topics/depression/index.shtml (accessed September 30, 2020).

NIMH. 2020f. Eating disorders. Bethesda, MD. https://www.nimh.nih.gov/health/topics/eating-disorders/index.shtml (accessed September 30, 2020).

NIMH. 2020g. Glossary. Bethesda, MD. https://www.nimh.nih.gov/health/topics/schizophrenia/raise/glossary.shtml (accessed January 5, 2021).

NIMH. 2020h. Mental illness. Bethesda, MD. https://www.nimh.nih.gov/health/statistics/mental-illness.shtml (accessed January 5, 2021).

NIMH. 2020i. Obsessive-compulsive disorder. Bethesda, MD. https://www.nimh.nih.gov/health/topics/obsessive-compulsive-disorder-ocd/index.shtml (accessed September 30, 2020).

NIMH. 2020j. Schizophrenia. Bethesda, MD. https://www.nimh.nih.gov/health/topics/schizophrenia/index.shtml (accessed September 30, 2020).

NIMH. 2020k. Suicide. Bethesda, MD. https://www.nimh.nih.gov/health/statistics/suicide.shtml (accessed December 15, 2020).

Nivet, M. A. 2015. A diversity 3.0 update: Are we moving the needle enough? *Academic Medicine* 90(12):1591-1593.

NMHA (National Mental Health Association). 1998. Depression in African Americans is not "just the blues." Arlington, VA.

Nobleza, D., J. Hagenbaugh, S. Blue, A. Stepchin, M. Vergare, and C. A. Pohl. 2018. The use of telehealth by medical and other health professional students at a college counseling center. *Journal of College Student Psychotherapy* 33(4):275-289.

Nock, M. K., G. Borges, E. J. Bromet, C. B. Cha, R. C. Kessler, and S. Lee. 2008. Suicide and suicidal behavior. *Epidemiologic Reviews* 30(1):133-154.

Núñez, A.-M., S. Hurtado, and E. Calderón Galdeano, eds. 2015. *Hispanic-serving institutions: Advancing research and transformative practices*. New York: Routledge.

O'Hanlon, C. E., A. M. Kranz, M. DeYoreo, A. Mahmud, C. L. Damberg, and J. Timbie. 2019. Access, quality, and financial performance of rural hospitals following health system affiliation. *Health Affairs* 38(12):2095-2104.

Obar, J. A., and A. Oeldorf-Hirsch. 2020. The biggest lie on the Internet: Ignoring the privacy policies and terms of service policies of social networking services. *Information, Communication and Society* 23(1):128-147.

Obermeyer, Z., B. Powers, C. Vogeli, and S. Mullainathan. 2019. Dissecting racial bias in an algorithm used to manage the health of populations. *Science* 366(6464):447-453.

Offer, D., K. I. Howard, K. A. Schonert, and E. Ostrov. 1991. To whom do adolescents turn for help? Differences between disturbed and nondisturbed adolescents. *Journal of the American Academy of Child and Adolescent Psychiatry* 30(4):623-630.

Okanagan charter: An international charter for health promoting universities and colleges. 2015. An outcome of the International Conference on Health Promoting Universities and Colleges, VII International Congress, Kelowna, British Columbia.

Ong, M., C. Wright, L. Espinosa, and G. Orfield. 2011. Inside the double bind: A synthesis of empirical research on undergraduate and graduate women of color in science, technology, engineering, and mathematics. *Harvard Educational Review* 81(2):172-209.

OPA (Office of Population Affairs). 2020. Adolescent health. Washington, DC: Department of Health and Human Services. https://opa.hhs.gov/adolescent-health?adolescent-development/mental-health/adolescent-mental-health-basics/common-disorders/index.html (accessed September 30, 2020).

Ort, S. 2020. The Carolina Covenant™: A low-income student financing initiative at the University of North Carolina at Chapel Hill. http://forum.mit.edu/wp-content/uploads/2017/06/Ford0604.pdf (accessed November 19, 2020).

Othman, N., F. Ahmad, C. El Morr, and P. Ritvo. 2019. Perceived impact of contextual determinants on depression, anxiety and stress: A survey with university students. *International Journal of Mental Health Systems* 13, article 17. https://doi.org/10.1186/s13033-019-0275-x.

Panchal, N., R. Kamal, K. Orgera, C. Cox, R. Garfield, L. Hamel, C. Muñana, and P. Chidambaram. 2020. *The implications of COVID-19 for mental health and substance use.* Washington, DC: Kaiser Family Foundation.

Panger, G., J. Tryon, and A. Smith. 2014. *Graduate student happiness and well-being report.* Berkeley: University of California.

Pannett, R. 2020. Coronavirus squeezes universities' finances as foreign students stay home. *Wall Street Journal*, March 29.

Parcover, J., M. J. Coiro, E. Finglass, and E. Barr. 2018. Effects of a brief mindfulness-based group intervention on college students. *Journal of College Student Psychotherapy* 32(4):312-329.

Parmelli, E., G. Flodgren, F. Beyer, N. Baillie, M. E. Schaafsma, and M. P. Eccles. 2011. The effectiveness of strategies to change organisational culture to improve healthcare performance: A systematic review. *Implementation Science* 6(1):33. doi: 10.1002/14651858.CD008315.pub2.

Păsărelu, C. R., G. Andersson, L. Bergman Nordgren, and A. Dobrean. 2017. Internet-delivered transdiagnostic and tailored cognitive behavioral therapy for anxiety and depression: A systematic review and meta-analysis of randomized controlled trials. *Cognitive Behaviour Therapy* 46(1):1-28.

Pedrelli, P., M. Nyer, A. Yeung, C. Zulauf, and T. Wilens. 2015. College students: Mental health problems and treatment considerations. *Academic Psychiatry* 39(5):503-511.

Perez, W., R. Espinoza, K. Ramos, H. M. Coronado, and R. Cortes. 2009. Academic resilience among undocumented Latino students. *Hispanic Journal of Behavioral Sciences* 31(2):149-181.

Perron, B. E., I. D. Grahovac, J. S. Uppal, M. T. Granillo, J. Shutter, and C. A. Porter. 2011. Supporting students in recovery on college campuses: Opportunities for student affairs professionals. *Journal of Student Affairs Research and Practice* 48(1):47-64.

Pfund, C., J. L. Branchaw, and J. Handelsman. 2015. *Entering mentoring.* 2nd ed. New York: W. H. Freeman.

Pinder-Amaker, S., and C. Bell. 2012. A bioecological systems approach for navigating the college mental health crisis. *Harvard Review of Psychiatry* 20(4):174-188.

Plaskett, S., D. Bali, M. J. Nakkula, and J. Harris. 2018. Peer mentoring to support first-generation low-income college students. *Phi Delta Kappan* 99(7):47-51.

Plimb, J. L., K. A. Bush, and S. E. Kersevich. 2016. Trauma-sensitive schools: An evidence-based approach. *School Social Work Journal* 40(2):37-60.

Pluhar, E., C. McCracken, K. L. Griffith, M. A. Christino, D. Sugimoto, and W. P. Meehan, III. 2019. Team sport athletes may be less likely to suffer anxiety or depression than individual sport athletes. *Journal of Sports Science and Medicine* 18(3):490-496.

PNPI (Postsecondary National Policy Institute). 2020a. First-generation students in higher education. Washington, DC. https://pnpi.org/first-generation-students/.

PNPI. 2020b. Post-traditional students. Washington, DC. https://pnpi.org/post-traditional-students (accessed September 30, 2020).

Poleman, W., N. Jenks-Jay, and J. Byrne. 2019. Nested networks: Transformational change in higher education. *Sustainability* 12(2):97-99.

Posselt, J. R. 2016. *Graduate student mental health in the United States.* Paper presented at the fall retreat of the National Academy of Education, Washington, DC.

Posselt, J. R. 2018a. Normalizing struggle: Dimensions of faculty support for doctoral students and implications for persistence and well-being. *Journal of Higher Education* 89(6):988-1013.

Posselt, J. R. 2018b. Rigor and support in racialized learning environments: The case of graduate education. *New Directions for Higher Education* 2018(181):59-70.

Posselt, J. R. 2020. *Equity in science: Representation, culture, and the dynamics of change in graduate education.* Palo Alto, CA: Stanford University Press.

Post, L., and M. Kelley. 2018. Student-athlete mental health. Pp. 439-448 in *Student mental health: A guide for psychiatrists, psychologists, and leaders serving in higher education,* L. W. Roberts, ed. Washington, DC: American Psychiatric Association.

Primm, A. B. 2019. The community college imperative: Designing solutions to promote the mental health of students. Steve Fund blog, January 10. Providence, RI. https://www.stevefund.org/blog-community-college-mental-health-solutions/ (accessed January 5, 2021).

Rasheem, S., A.-S. Alleman, D. Mushonga, D. Anderson, and H. F. Ofahengaue Vakalahi. 2018. Mentor-shape: Exploring the mentoring relationships of Black women in doctoral programs. *Mentoring and Tutoring: Partnership in Learning* 26(1):50-69.

Ray, M. E., J. M. Coon, A. A. Al-Jumaili, and M. Fullerton. 2019. Quantitative and qualitative factors associated with social isolation among graduate and professional health science students. *American Journal of Pharmaceutical Education* 83(7):6983.

Read, J. P., P. Ouimette, J. White, C. Colder, and S. Farrow. 2011. Rates of DSM–IV–TR trauma exposure and posttraumatic stress disorder among newly matriculated college students. *Psychological Trauma: Theory, Research, Practice, and Policy* 3(2):148-156.

Read, J. P., C. R. Colder, J. E. Merrill, P. Ouimette, J. White, and A. Swartout. 2012. Trauma and posttraumatic stress symptoms predict alcohol and other drug consequence trajectories in the first year of college. *Journal of Consulting and Clinical Psychology* 80(3):426-439.

Reddick, R. J., and K. O. Pritchett. 2015. "I don't want to work in a world of whiteness": White faculty and their developmental relationships with Black students. *Journal of the Professoriate* 8(1):54-84.

Reynolds, J., and S. Cruise. 2020. Factors that influence persistence among undergraduate students: An analysis of the impact of socioeconomic status and first-generation students. *Interchange: A Quarterly Review of Education* 51(2):199-206.

Rojas-Sosa, D. 2016. The denial of racism in Latina/o students' narratives about discrimination in the classroom. *Discourse and Society* 27(1):69-94.

Rotenstein, L. S., M. A. Ramos, M. Torre, J. B. Segal, M. J. Peluso, C. Guille, S. Sen, and D. A. Mata. 2016. Prevalence of depression, depressive symptoms, and suicidal ideation among medical students: A systematic review and meta-analysis. *JAMA* 316(21):2214-2236.

Ryu, D., and A. L. Thompson. 2018. Students of color. Pp. 399-403 in *Student mental health: A guide for psychiatrists, psychologists, and leaders serving in higher education,* L. W. Roberts, ed. Washington, DC: American Psychiatric Association.

SAMHSA (Substance Abuse and Mental Health Services Administration) and NSDUH. 2014. *Results from the 2012 National Survey on Drug Use and Health: Detailed tables.* Rockville, MD. https://www.samhsa.gov/data/report/results-2012-national-survey-drug-use-and-health-detailed-tables-table-contents (accessed December 15, 2020).

SAMHSA. 2018. *Behavioral health among college students information and resource kit.* Rockville, MD. https://store.samhsa.gov/product/Behavioral-Health-Among-College-Students-Information-and-Resource-Kit/SMA19-5052.

SAMHSA. 2019. *Results from the 2018 National Survey on Drug Use and Health: Detailed tables.* Rockville, MD. https://www.samhsa.gov/data/report/2018-nsduh-detailed-tables (accessed September 30, 2020).

SAMHSA. 2020a. Historically Black Colleges and Universities Center for Excellence in Behavioral Health. Rockville, MD. https://www.samhsa.gov/historically-black-colleges-universities-center-excellence-behavioral-health (accessed December 8, 2020).

SAMHSA. 2020b. Mental health and substance use disorders. Rockville, MD. https://www.samhsa.gov/find-help/disorders (accessed September 30, 2020).

Samuels, M. 2019. Professor launches "return on investment" tool for college student mental health. April 22. Boston, MA: Boston University School of Public Health. https://www.bu.edu/sph/news/articles/2019/professor-launches-return-on-investment-tool-for-college-student-mental-health (accessed December 15, 2020).

Sarikakis, K., and L. Winter. 2017. Social media users' legal consciousness about privacy. *Social Media + Society* 3(1):2056305117695325.

Scheffler, R. M., S. P. Hinshaw, S. Modrek, and P. Levine. 2007. The global market for ADHD medications. *Health Affairs* 26(2):450-457.

Schein, E. H. (2010). *Organizational culture and leadership* (4th ed.) (pp. 299–314). San Francisco, CA: Jossey-Bass.

Schifrin, M., and C. Coudriet. 2019. Dawn of the dead: For hundreds of the nation's private colleges, it's merge or perish. *Forbes*, November 27.

Schneider, B., M. Ehrhart, and W. Macey. 2012. Organizational Climate and Culture. *Annual review of psychology.* 64. 10.1146/annurev-psych-113011-143809.

Schulenberg, J. E., L. D. Johnston, P. M. O'Malley, J. G. Bachman, R. A. Miech, and M. E. Patrick. 2019. *Monitoring the future national survey results on drug use, 1975–2018: Volume II, college students and adults ages 19–60.* Ann Arbor: University of Michigan Institute for Social Research. http://www.monitoringthefuture.org/pubs/monographs/mtf-vol2_2018.pdf (accessed September 30, 2020).

Schweitzer, R., M. Klayich, and J. McLean. 1995. Suicidal ideation and behaviours among university students in Australia. *Australian and New Zealand Journal of Psychiatry* 29(3):473-479.

Scribner, R., K. Mason, K. Theall, N. Simonsen, S. K. Schneider, L. G. Towvim, and W. DeJong. 2008. The contextual role of alcohol outlet density in college drinking. *Journal of Studies on Alcohol and Drugs* 69(1):112-120.

Selingo, J. J. 2015. *The view from the top: What presidents think about financial sustainability, student outcomes, and the future of higher education.* Washington, DC: The Chronicle of Higher Education.

Sen, S., H. R. Kranzler, J. H. Krystal, H. Speller, G. Chan, J. Gelernter, and C. Guille. 2010. A prospective cohort study investigating factors associated with depression during medical internship. *Archives of General Psychiatry* 67(6):557-565.

Settles, I. H., L. M. Cortina, J. Malley, and A. J. Stewart. 2006. The climate for women in academic science: The good, the bad, and the changeable. *Psychology of Women Quarterly*, 30, 47-58.

SGMRO (Sexual and Gender Minority Research Office). 2020. Bethesda, MD: National Institutes of Health. https://dpcpsi.nih.gov/sgmro (accessed December 9, 2020).

Shah, R., N. Eshel, and L. McGlynn. 2018. Lesbian, gay, bisexual, transgender, and queer/questioning students. Pp. 411-424 in *Student mental health: A guide for psychiatrists, psychologists, and leaders serving in higher education*, L. W. Roberts, ed. Washington, DC: American Psychiatric Association.

Shankar, N. L., and C. L. Park. 2016. Effects of stress on students' physical and mental health and academic success. *International Journal of School and Educational Psychology* 4(1):5-9.

Shrivastava, A., M. Johnston, and M. Tsuang. 2011. Cannabis use and cognitive dysfunction. *Indian Journal of Psychiatry* 53(3):187-191.

Slavin, S. 2018. Medical student mental health: Challenges and opportunities. *Medical Science Educator* 28(1):13-15.

Slavin, S. 2019. Reflections on a decade leading a medical student well-being initiative. *Academic Medicine* 94(6):771-774.

Slavin, S. J., and J. T. Chibnall. 2016. Finding the why, changing the how: Improving the mental health of medical students, residents, and physicians. *Academic Medicine* 91(9):1194-1196.

Slavin, S. J., D. L. Schindler, and J. T. Chibnall. 2014. Medical student mental health 3.0: Improving student wellness through curricular changes. *Academic Medicine* 89(4):573-577.

Slopen, N., J. P. Shonkoff, M. A. Albert, H. Yoshikawa, A. Jacobs, R. Stoltz, and D. R. Williams. 2016. Racial disparities in child adversity in the U.S.: Interactions with family immigration history and income. *American Journal of Preventive Medicine* 50(1):47-56.

Slusser, W. M., H. Malan, and T. G. Watson, M. S. Goldstein. 2018. Collective impact for health and wellbeing. Stanford Social Innovation Review, March 12. https://ssir.org/articles/entry/collective_impact_for_health_and_wellbeing (accessed April 28, 2020).

Slutske, W. S. 2005. Alcohol use disorders among U.S. college students and their non-college-attending peers. *Archives of General Psychiatry* 62(3):321-327.

Snyder, T. D., C. de Brey, and S. A. Dillow. 2019. *Digest of education statistics 2018.* NCES 2020-009. Washington, DC: National Center for Education Statistics, Institute of Education Sciences, Department of Education.

Sohn, H. 2017. Racial and ethnic disparities in health insurance coverage: Dynamics of gaining and losing coverage over the life-course. *Population Research and Policy Review* 36(2):181-201.

Son, C., S. Hegde, A. Smith, X. Wang, F. Sasangohar. 2020. Effects of COVID-19 on college students' mental health in the United States: Interview survey study. *Journal of Medical Internet Research* 22(9):e21279.

Sontag-Padilla, L., M. Stephen Dunbar, R. Seelam, C. A. Kase, C. M. Setodji, and B. D. Stein. 2018a. California community college faculty and staff help address student mental health issues. *RAND Health Quarterly* 8(2):4.

Sontag-Padilla, L., M. S. Dunbar, F. Ye, C. Kase, R. Fein, S. Abelson, R. Seelam, and B. D. Stein. 2018b. Strengthening college students' mental health knowledge, awareness, and helping behaviors: The impact of Active Minds, a peer mental health organization. *Journal of the American Academy of Child and Adolescent Psychiatry* 57(7):500-507.

Spalter-Roth, R., and W. Erskine. 2007. *Race and ethnicity in the sociology pipeline.* Washington, DC: American Sociological Association.

Spitzer, R. L., K. Kroenke, and J. B. Williams. 1999. Validation and utility of a self-report version of PRIME-MD: The PHQ primary care study. Primary Care Evaluation of Mental Disorders. Patient Health Questionnaire. *JAMA* 282(18):1737-1744.

SPRC (Suicide Prevention Resource Center). 2004. *Promoting mental health and preventing suicide in college and university settings.* Newton, MA: Education Development Center.

SPRC. 2020. A comprehensive approach to suicide prevention. Oklahoma City, OK. http://www.sprc.org/effective-prevention/comprehensive-approach (accessed January 5, 2021).

Stamarski, C. S., and L. S. Son Hing. 2015. Gender inequalities in the workplace: The effects of organizational structures, processes, practices, and decision makers' sexism. *Frontiers in Psychology*, 6, Article 1400.

Startz, D. 2020. Coronavirus poses serious financial risks to U.S. universities. Brown Center Chalkboard, April 21. Washington, DC: Brookings Institution.

Stephens, N. M., M. G. Hamedani, and M. Destin. 2014. Closing the social-class achievement gap: A difference-education intervention improves first-generation students' academic performance and all students' college transition. *Psychological Science* 25(4):943-953.

Steve Fund. 2020. *Adapting and innovating to promote mental health and emotional well-being of young people of color: COVID-19 and beyond.* New York. https://www.stevefund.org/wp-content/uploads/2020/09/CRISIS-RESPONSE-TASK-FORCE-STEVE-FUND-REPORT.pdf (accessed December 9, 2020).

Steve Fund and Jed Foundation. 2017. *The equity in mental health framework.* New York: Steve Fund.

Stuart, G., and C. Lee. 2013. *Mental health promotions focus groups report.* Austin, TX: Counseling and Mental Health Center.

Suárez-Orozco, C., D. Katsiaficas, O. Birchall, C. M. Alcantar, E. Hernandez, Y. Garcia, M. Michikyan, J. Cerda, and R. T. Teranishi. 2015. Undocumented undergraduates on college campuses: Understanding their challenges and assets and what it takes to make an undocufriendly campus. *Harvard Educational Review* 85(3):427-463.

SVA (Student Veterans of America). 2020. SVA history. Washington, DC. https://studentveterans.org/about/history/ (accessed September 24, 2020).

Syed, M., M. Azmitia, and C. R. Cooper. 2011. Identity and academic success among underrepresented ethnic minorities: An interdisciplinary review and integration. *Journal of Social Issues* 67(3):442-468.

Taylor, P. 2016. The demographic trends shaping American politics in 2016 and beyond. *FactTank: News in the Numbers*, January 27. Washington, DC: Pew Research Center. https://www.pewresearch.org/fact-tank/2016/01/27/the-demographic-trends-shaping-american-politics-in-2016-and-beyond/.

Thielking, M. 2017. A dangerous wait: Colleges can't meet soaring student needs for mental health care. *STAT*, February 6.

Topham, P., and N. Moller. 2011. New students' psychological well-being and its relation to first-year academic performance in a UK university. *Counselling and Psychotherapy Research* 11(3):196-203.

Travia, R. M., J. G. Larcus, S. Andes, and P. G. Gomes. 2019. *Framing well-being in a college campus setting.* Silver Spring, MD: American College Health Foundation.

Trice, H. M., and J. M. Beyer. 1993. *The cultures of work organizations.* Englewood Cliffs, NJ: Prentice-Hall, Inc.

Turk, J., M. C. Soler, H. M. Chessman, and Á. Gonzalez. 2020. *College and university presidents respond to COVID-19: 2020 fall term survey, part II.* Washington, DC: American Council on Education. https://www.acenet.edu/Documents/Presidents-Respond-COVID-19-Fall2020-Part-Two.pdf (accessed December 15, 2020).

Turner, J. C., E. V. Leno, and A. Keller. 2013. Causes of mortality among American college students: A pilot study. *Journal of College Student Psychotherapy* 27(1):31-42.

Turner, S., and J. Bound. 2003. Closing the gap or widening the divide: The effects of the G.I. bill and World War II on the educational outcomes of Black Americans. *Journal of Economic History* 63(1):145-177.

UNC (University of North Carolina). 2020. Carolina Covenant. Chapel Hill. https://studentaid.unc.edu/incoming/what-aid-is-available/carolina-covenant/ (accessed November 19, 2020).

U.S. Congress. 2004. Garrett Lee Smith Memorial Act. Washington, DC. https://www.congress.gov/bill/108th-congress/senate-bill/2634 (accessed December 14, 2020).

UT (University of Texas at Austin). 2019. *Texas well-being: Promoting well-being in UT learning environments.* Austin, TX. https://www.cmhc.utexas.edu/wellbeing/images/guidebook.pdf (accessed January 5, 2021).

Van Brunt, B., and ACCA PAPA Committee. 2010. *The preparation and role of college counselors.* Alexandria, VA: American Counseling Association.

Velazquez, C. E., K. E. Pasch, M. N. Laska, K. Lust, M. Story, and E. P. Ehlinger. 2011. Differential prevalence of alcohol use among 2-year and 4-year college students. *Addictive Behaviors* 36(12):1353-1356.

Verschelden, C. 2017. *Bandwidth recovery: Helping students reclaim cognitive resources lost to poverty, racism, and social marginalization.* Sterling, VA: Stylus Publishing.

Volkow, N. D., J. M. Swanson, A. E. Evins, L. E. DeLisi, M. H. Meier, R. Gonzalez, M. A. Bloomfield, H. V. Curran, and R. Baler. 2016. Effects of cannabis use on human behavior, including cognition, motivation, and psychosis: A review. *JAMA Psychiatry* 73(3):292-297.

Wadsworth, B. C., M. L. Hecht, and E. Jung. 2008. The role of identity gaps, discrimination, and acculturation in international students' educational satisfaction in American classrooms. *Communication Education* 57(1):64-87.

Walsh, K., H. M. Zinzow, C. L. Badour, K. J. Ruggiero, D. G. Kilpatrick, and H. S. Resnick. 2016. Understanding disparities in service seeking following forcible versus drug- or alcohol-facilitated/incapacitated rape. *Journal of Interpersonal Violence* 31(14):2475-2491.

Walton, G. M., and G. L. Cohen. 2011. A brief social-belonging intervention improves academic and health outcomes of minority students. *Science* 331(6023):1447-1451.

Wang, R. S., and S. V. Joshi. 2018. First-generation college students. Pp. 389-398 in *Student mental health: A guide for psychiatrists, psychologists, and leaders serving in higher education*, L. W. Roberts, ed. Washington, DC: American Psychiatric Association.

Wechsler, H., J. E. Lee, J. Gledhill-Hoyt, and T. F. Nelson. 2001. Alcohol use and problems at colleges banning alcohol: Results of a national survey. *Journal of Studies on Alcohol and Drugs* 62(2):133-141.

Weil, A. R. 2014. It takes a community. *Health Affairs* 33(11):1886.

Weiner, S. 2018. Addressing the escalating psychiatrist shortage. February 12. Washington, DC: Association of American Medical Colleges. https://www.aamc.org/news-insights/addressing-escalating-psychiatrist-shortage (accessed August 31, 2020).

Weitzman, E. R., A. Folkman, M. P. Folkman, and H. Wechsler. 2003. The relationship of alcohol outlet density to heavy and frequent drinking and drinking-related problems among college students at eight universities. *Health and Place* 9(1):1-6.

Wilbur, T. G., and V. J. Roscigno. 2016. First-generation disadvantage and college enrollment/completion. *Socius* 2:2378023116664351.

Wilson, C., and L. A. Cariola. 2019. LGBTQI+ youth and mental health: A systematic review of qualitative research. *Adolescent Research Review* 5:187-211.

Wirt, L. G., and A. J. Jaeger. 2014. Seeking to understand faculty-student interaction at community colleges. *Community College Journal of Research and Practice* 38(11):980-994.

Wong, W. C. W., L. Song, C. See, S. T. H. Lau, W. H. Sun, K. W. Y. Choi, and J. Tucker. 2020. Using crowdsourcing to develop a peer-led intervention for safer dating app use: Pilot study. *JMIR Formative Research* 4(4):e12098.

Xiao, H., D. M. Carney, S. J. Youn, R. A. Janis, L. G. Castonguay, J. A. Hayes, and B. D. Locke. 2017. Are we in crisis? National mental health and treatment trends in college counseling centers. *Psychological Services* 14(4):407-415.

Zhu, Y. 2017. Pro-smoking information scanning using social media predicts young adults' smoking behavior. *Computers in Human Behavior* 77:19-24.

Appendix A

Committee Biographies

Alan I. Leshner is Chief Executive Officer, Emeritus, of the American Association for the Advancement of Science (AAAS) and former Executive Publisher of the *Science* family of journals. Before this position, Dr. Leshner was Director of the National Institute on Drug Abuse at the National Institutes of Health. He also served as Deputy Director and Acting Director of the National Institute of Mental Health, and in several roles at the National Science Foundation. Before joining the government, Dr. Leshner was Professor of Psychology at Bucknell University. Dr. Leshner is an elected fellow of AAAS, the American Academy of Arts and Sciences, the National Academy of Public Administration, and many others. He is a member and served on the governing Council of the National Academy of Medicine (formerly the Institute of Medicine) of the National Academies of Sciences, Engineering, and Medicine. He served two terms on the National Science Board, appointed first by President Bush and then reappointed by President Obama. Dr. Leshner received Ph.D. and M.S. degrees in physiological psychology from Rutgers University and an A.B. in psychology from Franklin and Marshall College. He has been awarded seven honorary Doctor of Science degrees.

Chris Brownson, a licensed psychologist, is Associate Vice President for Student Affairs, Director of the Counseling and Mental Health Center, and a Clinical Associate Professor in the Counseling Psychology Program at The University of Texas (UT) at Austin. His portfolio also includes oversight of University Health Services, the Longhorn Wellness Center, and the Center for Students in Recovery. He is a faculty fellow of the Institute of Urban Policy and Research Analysis. Dr. Brownson is the director of the National Research Consortium of Counseling Centers in Higher Education, and his research interests include college student suicide prevention, collaborative care models in primary care, and the intersection of mental health and academic success. As a consultant, he is regularly involved in program reviews and evaluations of college and university counseling centers and health centers. He is a past president of the Texas University and College Counseling Center Director's Association. He is past chair of the Higher Education Mental Health Alliance, the Section on College and University Counseling Centers of the American Psychological Association's Division of Counseling Psychology, and the Mental Health Section of the American College Health Association. He is a past member of the Board of Directors of the American College Health Association. He co-developed the Integrated Health Program at UT, which utilizes behavioral medicine and mindfulness-based interventions in a primary care environment, promoting collaboration between medical and mental health providers. In 2014, Dr. Brownson was appointed as a Chancellor's Health Fellow at UT System and he currently leads a $6 million project implementing various mental health, student safety, and alcohol-related initiatives at the 14 academic and health institutions of the UT System. In 2016, he received the Texas Impact Award from Mental Health America Texas. Dr. Brownson has given over 90 invited addresses or professional conference presentations on topics such as behavioral health and primary care, smoking cessation, the roles of professional organizations within college mental health, collegiate recovery, college student mental health, college student suicide and suicide prevention, and the intersection of well-being and academic success. He has published more than 30 articles, book chapters, and opinion pieces on the role of research in college counseling centers, integration of mental health and primary care, group counseling, fatherhood, college student suicide prevention, the intersection of identity and suicidal behavior, and academic success. Dr. Brownson has his Ph.D. in counseling psychology and quantitative methods, with a specialization in psychometrics, from The University of Texas at Austin, where he also received his M.A. and his B.A.

Gerard Clancy, MD, serves as the Senior Associate Dean for External Affairs and Clinical Professor of Psychiatry in the University of Iowa's Carver College of Medicine. He is a graduate of the University of Iowa with degrees in biochemistry and medicine, with Alpha Omega Alpha Honors, an American Heart Association Molecular Biology Research Fellowship and Residency Training as a Psychiatrist, with service as the Chief Resident. He served as a Flight Surgeon in the United States Air Force with specialty training in aerospace medicine, survival medicine and hostage negotiations. He is also a graduate of Harvard University programs in health policy and management and non-profit financial stewardship. Dr. Clancy has published peer-reviewed manuscripts and presented across the world on molecular biology, addiction, chronic mental illness, health disparities, and health systems transformation. He has received numerous teaching awards including the 2016 Crimson Apple Award for Teaching Excellence and the 2018 Outstanding Teacher Award in the University of Oklahoma—University of Tulsa

School of Community Medicine. In 2017, he received the National Brodie Medical Education Scholar Award. Dr. Clancy has been a founding Dean of a college twice. In 2008, he led the establishment of the University of Oklahoma—University of Tulsa School of Community Medicine. In 2015, he led the establishment of the University of Tulsa's Oxley College of Health Sciences. He led the creation of numerous clinical and education programs including outreach mental health services for the homeless, school-based clinics, the Bedlam Evening Clinics for the uninsured, the Wayman Tisdale Clinic in North Tulsa, and Tulsa's Albert Schweitzer Fellowship. Dr. Clancy was been deeply involved in the Tulsa Community. He was the team leader for the Lewin Study, which discovered the 14-year difference in life expectancy between north and south Tulsa. He was again the team leader in discovering a 27-year difference in life expectancy for those with chronic mental illness in the Tulsa region. In 2011 he was the Chairman of the Board of the Tulsa Regional Chamber of Commerce. In 2015, he was the Chairman of the Board of the Tulsa Area United Way. Over his 12 years as a university president at the University of Tulsa and the University of Oklahoma, Tulsa, Dr. Clancy has raised more than $510 million in support of student scholarships, 72 endowed chairs, 250,000 sq. ft. of new facilities, and a host of new education programs. Dr. Clancy has received the Distinguished Alumni Award for Early Achievement from the University of Iowa Carver College of Medicine and the Distinguished Alumni Award from the University of Iowa. He was Tulsa People magazine's 2009 Tulsan of the Year, and in 2016 he received the Heart of Henry Zarrow Humanitarian Award. The National Alliance on Mental Illness presented Dr. Clancy with the Exemplary Psychiatrist Award and twice their Public Service Award. In January, Dr. Clancy received the 2020 National University President of the Year Award at the Student Veterans of America National Conference in Los Angeles for his work on student veteran well-being and academic success.

Bonnie Duran, DrPH, is a Professor in the Schools of Social Work and Public Health at the University of Washington (UW), in Seattle. After completing her doctoral degree at the University of California Berkeley, she has worked in public health and social care research, education and practice with a focus on Native Americans/Indigenous peoples and other communities of color for more than 35 years. Dr. Duran has conducted primary and secondary data analysis studies of mental disorder prevalence, risk and protective factors, victimization, and treatment seeking/ barriers to care among people attending Indian Health Service (IHS) facilities and probability samples from the largest rural Tribal Nations in the United States. In partnership with communities, she has adapted and developed Indigenous interventions for system level, community, and individual health and wellbeing. Another aspect of Dr. Duran's empirical work is the development of indigenous theory and Community-Based Participatory Research (CBPR) methods. She has pioneered the development and application of CBPR and other forms of Community-Engaged Research (CEnR) and has helped to articulate and disseminate the theory of Historical Trauma. For the past 12 years she has worked in close partnership with the American Indian Higher Education Consortium and Tribal College faculty, staff, and students to conduct Indigenous culture-centered epidemiology and interventions research to enhance college success. Dr. Duran is currently co-chair of the Coronavirus Prevention Network Indigenous Expert Panel and is on a UW COVID-19 Vaccine Trial research team. The overall goals of her research and practice are to work in partnership with communities to design treatment and prevention efforts that are effective, empowering, and sustainable, and that have maximum public health impact. Dr. Duran is also a Buddhist Mindfulness practitioner and teacher. She teaches long and short retreats and advanced programs at the Insight Meditation Society (IMS) in Massachusetts and Spirit Rock Meditation Center (SRMC) in California and is on the SRMC Guiding Teachers Council.

Daniel Eisenberg is Professor of Health Policy and Management in the Fielding School of Public Health at the University of California (UC), Los Angeles. Previously he was a faculty member at University of Michigan from 2004-2020. His training is in economics (BA and PhD, Stanford University) and mental health services research (NIMH postdoc, UC Berkeley). His broad research goal is to improve understanding of how to invest effectively in the mental health of young people. He directs the Healthy Minds Network (HMN) for Research on Adolescent and Young Adult Mental Health (www.healthymindsnetwork.org). This research network administers the Healthy Minds Study, a national survey study of student mental health and related factors, and facilitates the development, testing, and dissemination of innovative programs and interventions for student mental health. He is currently writing a book about investments in children's mental health, in collaboration with Ramesh Raghavan.

Raynard S. Kington began his work as Head of School at Phillips Academy in Andover, Massachusetts, in July 2020. Prior to joining Andover, he served for 10 years as President of Grinnell College (2010-2020) and previously in a range of positions at the National Institutes of Health (NIH), including NIH Principal Deputy Director and NIH Acting Director, NIH Associate Director for Behavioral and Social Sciences Research, and Acting Director of the National Institute on Alcohol Abuse and Alcoholism. Before NIH he was a division director at the Centers for Disease Control and Prevention and served as Director of the National Health and Nutrition Examination Survey (NHANES). He has also been a Senior Scientist at the RAND Corporation and an Assistant Professor of Medicine at UCLA. He was elected to the Institute of Medicine (now, the National Academy of Medicine) in 2006. Dr. Kington attended the University of Michigan, where he received both his BS with distinction and his MD and completed his residency in Internal Medicine at Michael Reese Medical Center in Chicago. He was a Robert Wood Johnson Clinical Scholar at the University

of Pennsylvania where he completed his MBA with distinction and his PhD with
a concentration in Health Policy and Economics at the Wharton School and was
awarded a Fontaine Fellowship. He received his board certification in Internal
Medicine, Public Health and Preventive Medicine, and Geriatric Medicine. His
research has focused on the social determinants of health and more recently on
diversity in the scientific workforce.

Amy Lenhart is a licensed professional mental health counselor supervisor in
the state of Texas (LPC-S) and also is a Nationally Certified Counselor (NCC).
Ms. Lenhart has worked providing mental health counseling to students in the
community college setting for more than twenty years. Amy is currently serving
community college students in her twentieth year as a mental health counselor for
Collin College, and has previous work experience in a domestic violence agency.
Ms. Lenhart holds an MA in counseling and psychology in education, graduating
with honors. A strong believer in advocacy for students and college counseling, Amy has worked to promote awareness in her state and national leadership
roles. She is a past-president of the American College Counseling Association
(ACCA) becoming the first president elected from a community college. She has
also served as a member at large for ACCA. Ms. Lenhart was elected president
of the Texas College Counseling Association (TCCA) having previously held
the positions of senator and treasurer. She also chaired an ex officio committee
for TCCA that resulted in changes by the Southern Association of Colleges and
Schools in regard to specific language concerning college counseling standards.
Awards and honors include a leadership award from ACCA, the TCCA award for
Outstanding College Counselor, as well as a merit award from the Texas Career
Development Association. She has presented internationally, nationally, and in
her state on college counseling and mental health topics. She has been quoted by
The Straits Times, *The Chronicle of Higher Education*, and *Insight into Diversity*
for her expertise regarding mental health issues in the college setting. She is also
the co-author of a national research survey on college counseling.

Frances Leslie, professor of Pharmaceutical Sciences at the University of California Irvine (UCI), is a neuropharmacologist with a primary interest in the effects of drugs of abuse on the developing brain. She received her PhD from the
University of Aberdeen, Scotland, where she participated in landmark studies
on the identification and mechanism of action of enkephalin, the first endorphin
discovered. She has been continuously funded by the National Institutes of Health
and the UC Tobacco Related Disease Research Program since establishing her
laboratory in 1981. At UCI, she has also served as Associate Vice Chancellor
for Research from 1995-1998 and Director of an NIH-funded Transdisciplinary
Tobacco Use Center from 1999 to 2005. With a strong commitment to graduate
education, Dr. Leslie served as Dean of UCI Graduate Division from 2008 to
2019. In this capacity, she focused on building resources to attract and retain the

best and brightest graduate students and to prepare them for future leadership positions. She created the Diverse Educational Community and Doctoral Experience (DECADE) program, with initial support from a Department of Education FIPSE grant, to establish a diverse student learning community on the UCI campus. This program was subsequently institutionalized and expanded with a Department of Education Title III award to establish a model of graduate student mentoring of undergraduate students.

Ben Locke, PhD, is the Founder and Executive Director of the Center for Collegiate Mental Health (CCMH, a practice-research network of more than 600 institutions), the Senior Director of Counseling and Psychological Services at Penn State, and affiliate graduate faculty in both the Counseling and Clinical Psychology departments at Penn State. Dr. Locke presents and consults widely about college student mental health, and counseling center administration and has published dozens of peer-reviewed articles in the field. Dr. Locke has more than 20 years of clinical experience in a wide variety of settings including wilderness therapy, psychiatric hospitals, group homes, community mental health, and college counseling centers. He received his BA in psychology from the University of New Hampshire, and his MA, and PhD in counseling psychology from Boston College.

Gail Mattox currently serves as professor and chair of the department of psychiatry at the Morehouse School of Medicine (MSM). She is a diplomate of the American Board of Psychiatry and Neurology with board certification in psychiatry and sub-specialty board certification in child and adolescent psychiatry. She is a graduate of Meharry Medical College and completed psychiatry training at the Northwestern University Feinberg School of Medicine. Dr. Mattox is a Distinguished Life Fellow of the American Psychiatric Association and a Distinguished Life Fellow of the American Academy of Child and Adolescent Psychiatry. Dr. Mattox is also a member of Alpha Omega Alpha Medical Honor Society and the Arnold P. Gold Humanism in Medicine Honor Society. In addition to teaching, patient care, community service, and administrative duties, Dr. Mattox served as Project Director for more than 10 years for the National Historically Black Colleges and Universities (HBCU) Center for Excellence in Behavioral Health funded through a cooperative agreement from the Substance Abuse and Mental Health Services Administration (SAMHSA).

Maria A. Oquendo MD, PhD is the Ruth Meltzer Professor and Chairman of Psychiatry at University of Pennsylvania and Psychiatrist-in-Chief at the Hospital of the University of Pennsylvania. She is a graduate of Tufts University and attended Vagelos College of Physicians and Surgeons, Columbia University. She completed residency at Payne Whitney Clinic, New York Hospital, Weil-Cornell. Until 2016, she was Professor of Psychiatry and Vice Chairman for Education at Columbia. In 2017, she was elected to the National Academy of Medicine, one of the highest honors in medicine. Dr. Oquendo has used positron emission tomography and magnetic resonance imaging to map brain abnormalities in mood disorders and suicidal behavior. Her expertise ranges from psychopharmacology to global mental health. She has more than 400 peer-reviewed publications and an h-factor of 76 with more than 17,000 citations. Dr. Oquendo is Past President of the American Psychiatric Association (APA) and the International Academy of Suicide Research. She is President of the American College of Neuropsychopharmacology (ACNP) and of the American Foundation for Suicide Prevention's Board of Directors and has served on the National Institute of Mental Health's Advisory Council. She is a Fellow of the ACNP, APA, and American College of Psychiatrists (ACP). Dr. Oquendo is a member of Tufts University's Board of Trustees, serves on its Executive Committee, and chairs Tufts' Academic Affairs Committee. A recipient of multiple awards in the United States, Europe, and South America, most recently she was honored with the Virginia Kneeland Award for Distinguished Women in Medicine (Columbia University 2016), the Award for Mood Disorders Research (ACP 2017), the Alexandra Symonds Award (APA 2017), the APA's Research Award (2018), and the Dolores Shockley Award (ACNP 2018).

Stephanie Pinder-Amaker, PhD is Chief Diversity, Equity, and Inclusion Officer at McLean Hospital and Director, College Mental Health Program. Dr. Pinder-Amaker is also Assistant Professor of Psychology, Department of Psychiatry at Harvard Medical School. She has more than 25 years of experience in college student mental health treatment, administration, and policy. She is the founding director of McLean Hospital's College Mental Health Program, a unique initiative serving students from more than 200 institutions of higher education, providing student-focused treatment; consultation to students, parents, and college professionals, and nonprofits; and related research. Dr. Pinder-Amaker lectures and conducts workshops throughout the country on strengthening continuity of care, and on how to bolster communication between campus- and community-based systems, eliminate barriers to mental health treatment, and better support marginalized students. She is a member of the WHO World Mental Health International College Student Initiative and has published on the prevalence and distribution of mental disorders among college students and the integration of student concerns into traditional models of care. Dr. Pinder-Amaker has a BS from Duke University and a PhD in Clinical Psychology from Vanderbilt University.

Julie Posselt is an associate professor of higher education in the University of Southern California Rossier School of Education and was a 2015-2017 National Academy of Education/Spencer Foundation postdoctoral research fellow. Rooted in sociological and organizational theory, her research program uses mixed methods to examine institutionalized inequalities in higher education and organizational efforts aimed at reducing inequities and encouraging diversity. She focuses on selective sectors of higher education—graduate education, STEM fields, and elite undergraduate institutions—where longstanding practices and cultural norms are being negotiated to better identify talent and educate students in a changing society. She was the recipient of the 2018 American Educational Research Association's Early Career Award and the 2017 Association for the Study of Higher Education's Early Career/Promising Scholar Award. Her book, *Inside Graduate Admissions: Merit, Diversity, and Faculty Gatekeeping* (2016, Harvard University Press), was based on an award-winning ethnographic study of faculty judgment in 10 highly ranked doctoral programs in three universities. This work has led to thriving research-practice partnerships with universities, disciplinary societies, graduate schools and programs, and other associations that are re-examining how we evaluate students and scholars for key academic opportunities—and support those who are in the system. Partners include the University of California, American Physics Society, and the Council of Graduate Schools. Her current scholarship, funded by three grants from the National Science Foundation and one from the Mellon Foundation, examines movements for equity and inclusion in graduate education and the humanistic and physical science disciplines. Dr. Posselt recently completed a National Academy of Education postdoctoral fellowship for the first national study of graduate student mental health. This concurrent mixed methods project identified factors associated with depression and anxiety; investigated the roles of discrimination, competitiveness, and faculty support in graduate student wellbeing; and measured disparities within and across academic disciplines. Dr. Posselt earned her PhD from the University of Michigan.

Claire Sterk is Charles Howard Candler Professor at the Rollins School of Public Health at Emory University. A pioneering public health scholar, Dr. Sterk has served for the past two decades as a social scientist, academic leader, and administrator at Emory, most recently as University President and Provost/Executive Vice President of Academic Affairs. She is a globally renowned thought leader who has deepened our understanding of social and health disparities; addiction and infectious diseases, specifically HIV/AIDS; community engagement; and the importance of mentoring and empowering women leaders. She has held numerous leadership positions in professional organizations. Her academic publications include three books and more than 125 peer-reviewed articles. Her work is widely cited and has received $30 million in external research funding. She has lectured widely on key topics in public health and in higher education, including the student experience and student health and wellbeing. She is a strong advocate for collaboration and innovation and a champion for global engagement. Sterk also is a member of the American Academy of Arts and Sciences and the National Academy of Medicine. A native of the Netherlands, Dr. Sterk earned her PhD in sociology from Erasmus University (Rotterdam, the Netherlands), a doctorandus

8 the undergraduate degree from the Free University in Amsterdam.

Jeanie Tietjen, PhD is the director for the Institute for Trauma, Adversity, and Resilience in Higher Education at MassBay Community College, where she also serves as a professor of English. MassBay's Institute for Trauma, Adversity, and Resilience in Higher Education formalizes an ongoing recognition of complex interrelationships between trauma and learning in postsecondary education. It believes that every encounter area of the educational community—from pedagogy to campus safety, advising to financial aid, facilities to college policies and administration—can be informed by understanding the basics of the learning brain; the prevalence of trauma, adversity, and toxic stress; how resilience as skill can be encouraged through best practices and meaningful supports; and how evidence that just one relationship can powerfully bolster productive and resilient behaviors. Dr. Tietjen earned her PhD in English from Brandeis University.

Appendix B

Minority Serving Institutions

TABLE B-1 Historically Defined Minority Serving Institutions

MSI Type	Acronym	Federal Recognition	Federal Definition
Historically Black Colleges and Universities	HBCU	Higher Education Act of 1965	Any historically Black college or university established prior to 1964, whose principal mission was, and is, the education of Black Americans
Tribal Colleges and Universities	TCU	Tribally Controlled College or University Assistance Act of 1978	Institutions chartered by their respective Indian tribes through the sovereign authority of the tribes or by the federal government with the specific purpose to provide higher education opportunities to Native Americans through programs that are locally and culturally based, holistic, and supportive

TABLE B-2 Enrollment-Defined Minority Serving Institutions, as Defined by the U.S. Department of Education (NASEM, 2019a, Table 3-2)

MSI Type	Acronym	Federal Recognition	Federal Definition
Hispanic-Serving Institutions	HSIs	Higher Education Act of 1991	Institutions with 25 percent or more total undergraduate Hispanic full-time-equivalent student enrollment.
Alaska Native and Native Hawaiian-Serving Institutions	ANNHI	Higher Education Act of 1998	Alaska Native-Serving Institutions are institutions that have at least 20 percent Alaska Native students. Native Hawaiian-Serving Institutions are institutions that have at least 10 percent Native Hawaiian students. Collectively, these institutions are referred to as ANNHI institutions.
Asian American and Native American Pacific Islander-Serving Institutions	AANAPISI	College Cost Reduction and Access Act of 2007	Institutions that have at least 10 percent enrollment of Asian American Pacific Islander students.
Predominantly Black Institutions	PBI	Higher Education Opportunity Act of 2008	Institutions that have the following demographics: 1. at least 1,000 undergraduate students 2. at least 50 percent low-income or first-generation-to-college degree-seeking undergraduate enrollment 3. low per-full-time undergraduate expenditure in comparison with other institutions offering similar instruction 4. enroll at least 40 percent African American students
Native American-Serving, Nontribal Institutions	NASNTI	Native American-Serving, Nontribal Institutions	Institutions that have at least 10 percent enrollment of Native American students

Source: NASEM, 2019, Table 3-2.

Appendix C

Acronyms and Abbreviations

AACC	American Association of Community Colleges
AAMC	Association of American Medical Colleges
AANAPISI	Asian American and Native American Pacific Islander-Serving Institution
ACCA	American College Counseling Association
ACCA PAPA	American College Counseling Association Professional Advocacy and Public Awareness committee
ACE	American Council on Education
ACEs	Adverse Childhood Experiences
ACHA	American College Health Association
ACS	American Community Survey
ADA	Americans with Disabilities Act of 1990
ADAA	Anxiety and Depression Association of America
ADD	attention-deficit disorder
ADHD	attention-deficit/hyperactivity disorder
AIHEC	American Indian Higher Education Consortium
AMI	any mental illness
ANNHI	Alaska Native and Native Hawaiian-Serving Institution
ASD	autism spectrum disorder
AUCCCD	Association of University and College Counseling Center Directors
AUD	alcohol use disorder
BHEW	Board on Higher Education and Workforce
BIPOC	Black, Indigenous, and people of color
CAMHI	Child & Adolescent Mental Health Initiative program

CAT	computerized adaptive testing
CAT-MH	computerized adaptive testing-mental health suite
CCAPS	Counseling Center Assessment of Psychological Symptoms
CCMH	Center for Collegiate Mental Health
CDC	Centers for Disease Control and Prevention
CGS	Council of Graduate Schools
CLI	Clinical Load Index
College Fund	American Indian College Fund
CollegeAIM	College Alcohol Intervention Matrix
COVID-19	coronavirus disease of 2019
CRPs	collegiate recovery programs
DACA	Deferred Action for Childhood Arrivals
DOJ	U.S. Department of Justice
ED	U.S. Department of Education
FERPA	Family Educational Rights and Privacy Act of 1974
GAD	generalized anxiety disorder
G.I. Bill	Servicemen's Readjustment Act of 1944, commonly known as the G.I. Bill
GLSMA	Garrett Lee Smith Memorial Act of 2004
HBCU	Historically Black Colleges and Universities
HEA	Higher Education Act of 1991
HEMHA	Higher Education Mental Health Alliance
HHS	U.S. Department of Health and Human Services
HIPAA	Health Insurance Portability and Accountability Act of 1996
HIV	human immunodeficiency virus
HLC	Higher Learning Commission
HMD	Health and Medicine Division
HMN	Healthy Minds Network
HMS	Healthy Minds Study/Survey
HRC	Human Rights Campaign
HRSA	Health Resources and Services Administration
HIS	Hispanic-Serving Institution
IACS	International Accreditation of Counseling Services
KFF	Kaiser Family Foundation
LGBTQIAP+	Lesbian, Gay, Bisexual, Transgender, Questioning, Intersex, Asexual, Pansexual plus community
MD	Doctor of Medicine
MSI	Minority Serving Institution
MSM	men who have sex with men
MTF	Monitoring the Future general population survey
NASEM	National Academies of Sciences, Engineering, and Medicine
NASMHPD	National Association of State Mental Health Program Directors

NASNTI	Native American-Serving, Nontribal Institution
NCAA	National Collegiate Athletic Association
NCDJ	National Center on Disability and Journalism
NCES	National Center for Education Statistics
NCHA	National College Health Assessment
NIAAA	National Institute on Alcohol Abuse and Alcoholism
NIDA	National Institute on Drug Abuse
NIH	National Institutes of Health
NIMH	National Institute of Mental Health
NSC	National Student Clearinghouse
NSDUH	National Survey of Drug Use and Health
NSF	National Science Foundation
OCD	obsessive-compulsive disorder
PBI	Predominantly Black Institution
PHQ-9	Patient Health Questionnaire-9
PNPI	Postsecondary National Policy Institute
PTE	potentially traumatizing event
PTSD	post-traumatic stress disorder
RUI	Research in Undergraduate Institutions
SAMHSA	Substance Abuse and Mental Health Services Administration
SARS-CoV-2	severe acute respiratory syndrome coronavirus 2
SDS	standardized data set
SGM	sexual and gender minority
SGMRO	Sexual & Gender Minority Research Office
SPRC	Suicide Prevention Resource Center
SSM/V	student service members and veterans
STEM	sciences, technology, engineering, and mathematics
STEMM	sciences, technology, engineering, mathematics, and medicine
SUD	substance use disorder
SVA	Student Veterans of America
TBI	traumatic brain injury
TCU	Tribal Colleges and Universities
THC	tetrahydrocannabinol
UCOP	University of California Office of the President
WMH-ICS	World Mental Health International College Student initiative

Appendix D

The Rate of Student Death from Suicide from the Big Ten Counseling Centers: 2009-2018

Counseling Center, University of Illinois at Urbana-Champaign
Raquel Mendizábal Martell, Ph.D. & Matthew King, Ph.D.

Prepared for the Committee on Mental Health, Substance Use, and Wellbeing
of the National Academies of Sciences, Engineering, and Medicine

July 24, 2020

METHODOLOGY

Study Design

Silverman et al. (1997) conducted a comprehensive 10-year study at 13 Big Ten university campuses to get a more accurate understanding of deaths by suicide in college campuses. Silverman et al. (1997) collected data from 1980 to 1990, at which point the study stopped. In an effort to continue to understand suicide rates and trends in college campuses, the Big Ten university counseling centers decided to continue to collect data on deaths by suicides in their campuses. Data collection resumed in 2003 and it continues to be collected, with some data entered retrospectively and some data entered prospectively.

Representatives at the Big Ten universities counseling centers (e.g., directors, data analysts, designated staff) were asked to report all student deaths by suicide to a database. Each participating Big Ten universities counseling center sought research approval from their universities to participate in the study and contribute data. All schools have different methodologies by which they gather and contribute data to the database. Generally, representatives at the counseling centers received information about student deaths by suicide from other departments, such as the Office of Dean of Students, and then they entered relevant information into the database.

Time Frame

For the purpose of this report, data from the most recent 10 years were analyzed given that various universities could not verify the data on deaths by suicide for the early 2000s. Thus, the time frame for this report is September 1, 2009, to August 31, 2019. The current report uses an academic year time frame, which is defined as the 12-month period from September 1 to August 31. This reporting time frame is consistent to the time frame used by Silverman et al. (1997), which more closely aligns to academic calendars in university campuses, which is relevant as the population studied is college students.

While most universities entered data prospectively, some universities entered data for some years retrospectively. A few universities entered the study after its start, and thus entered some data retrospectively and some data prospectively as well. The Big Ten universities counseling centers consider the Suicide Registry an ongoing project and data continue to be collected.

Period of Exposure to Risk

The calculation of period of exposure to risk for the current analyses and report is consistent to Silverman et al. (1997). Specifically, for each academic year, the fall semester enrollment numbers for each university were added. Enrollment numbers were gathered using the public information available through each university's website. For universities for which only some of these data were available, general reported rates or percentages for each school were used to determine an approximate number of students for demographic information.

Definitions: Student Status and Suicide

The definitions of "student" and "student suicide" in this report were kept consistent to the definitions used by Silverman et al. (1997). A "student" is defined as an individual who was registered for credits as a full- or part-time student during the academic year in undergraduate or graduate programs in the main campuses at the Big Ten universities. A "student suicide" is a death by suicide that occurs by an individual who was a "student" as previously described within 6 months from being registered as an active student. The "6-month rule" accounts for student absences in which students are not actively registered for a short period of time such as summer months, academic leave, and medical leave (Silverman et al., 1997).

Consistent with Silverman et al. (1997), "suicide" is "a self-inflicted injury resulting in death" (p. 289). Representatives at each Big Ten counseling center identified a student death in their university as a "suicide" internally based on information they received of the incident. Student deaths for which cause was inconclusive based on the information representatives received (e.g., cause of death was considered unknown, accidental, or natural), were not included in the database or this study as they are not considered a death by suicide.

Confidentiality

The current study ensured adherence to proper research procedures and the confidentiality of personal information. All participating counseling center representatives sought the proper permissions in their respective universities (e.g., IRB approval) to contribute data.

To ensure that data were contributed in a secure way that would protect the identity and privacy of the students, all Big Ten universities were assigned a numerical "University Code" that they used to enter their data to the database rather than using the institution name. The data is stored in a secured database at the University of Illinois Counseling Center, which serves as the repository for this data. The raw database is only accessed by the study team. Data entered is not identifiable given that student names or initials are not entered. As such, the raw database does not have any first or last names, and universities have random numerical codes that have only been shared among the Big Ten counseling center representatives. All data are reported in aggregate form, and data were pooled when appropriate to ensure that data cannot be identified by school or to an individual.

Participating Universities

Thirteen Big Ten universities participated in and contributed data for the study. The 13 participating universities were located in the Midwest and Northeast in the United States in the following states: Illinois (Northwestern University, University of Illinois at Urbana – Champaign), Indiana (Indiana University, Purdue), Iowa (University of Iowa), Michigan (Michigan State, University of Michigan), Minnesota (University of Minnesota), Nebraska (University of Nebraska – Lincoln), New Jersey (Rutgers), Ohio (The Ohio State University), Pennsylvania (Pennsylvania State), Wisconsin (University of Wisconsin – Madison).

Data Sources

Enrollment and student population demographic data for participating Big Ten universities were obtained from public records and information published by each university through its website (e.g., Office of the Registrar website). Data from fall 2009 through fall 2018 were obtained. Enrollment and demographic data for most universities were readily available. Demographic and gender identity breakdowns for universities for which these data were not publicly and readily available were estimated using the information publicly available for each of those schools (e.g., percentages available).

Table D-1 summarizes enrollment numbers and student population demographic data. Academic class was used to classify academic parameters. There are two classifications: undergraduate (i.e., freshmen, sophomores, juniors, seniors, non-declared, or other undergraduate) and graduate (i.e., masters, doctorates, professionals, post-graduates). Gender identity is classified as male, female, and given the small numbers of reported students who identified as transgender or another gender, these numbers were pooled in the demographic information and in student suicide data with those whose gender was unknown under the category "Other." Racial identity is classified as Asian, Black, Hawaiian/ Pacific Islander, Hispanic, Native American, White, Multiracial, and Unknown. Given the small number of student suicides and students who identified as other than White, Asian, and Black, student suicides by a student who was Hawaiian/Pacific Islander, Hispanic, Native American, or Multiracial were classified as "Other." Given that some universities reported International/Foreign students as a racial group and other universities reported International/Foreign students separately and in addition to a racial category, analyses were run based on nationality with two classifications: International and Domestic.

Results

The total number of students across all Big Ten universities for the years (2009-2018) for which data were reported was about 4.8 million students (Table 1). The total number of deaths by suicide reported by the participating universities was 268, and the total number of deaths by suicide entered into the database by the participating universities was 231.

The overall average suicide rate per 100,000 students is 5.60 for the years 2009 to 2018 in the Big Ten college campuses. This is lower than the rate calculated by Silverman et al. (1997), which was 7.5/100,000. Specifically, there was a 25.3% decrease in the suicide rate in Big Ten universities in 30 years from 1980-1990 to 2009-2018.

The rate of 5.60 is also lower than the U.S. population national average suicide rate of 14.2/100,000 based on 2018 data from the National Center for Health Statistics (NCHS) at the Centers for Disease Control and Prevention (CDC; Hedegaard, Curtin, and Warner, 2020). The 5.60/100,000 rate in college

TABLE D-1 Demographic Profile of Campus Population at Big Ten Universities: 2009-2018

	Frequency	Percentage (%)
Gender Identity		
Female	2,330,169	48.68
Male	2,449,656	51.18
Unknown	6,579	0.14
Total	4,786,404	100
Race		
Asian	378,912	8.99
Black	215,944	5.12
Hawaiian/Pacific Islander	4,240	0.10
Hispanic	241,001	5.72
Native American	12,964	0.31
White	3,149,263	74.70
Multiracial	101,926	2.42
Unknown	111,366	2.64
Total	4,215,615	100
Nationality		
International	651,735	13.62
Domestic	4,134,669	86.38
Total	4,786,404	100
Class Standing		
Undergraduate	3,539,590	73.95
Graduate	1,246,814	26.05
Total	4,786,404	100

TABLE D-2 Student Deaths by Suicide at 13 Big Ten University Campuses (2009-2018)

	Frequency	Percentage (%)	Suicide Rate*	95% CI
Gender Identity				
Female	40	17.32	1.72	(1.23–2.34)
Male	156	67.53	6.37	(5.41–7.45)
Unknown/Other	35	15.15		
Total	231	100.0		
Race				
Asian	24	10.39	6.33	(4.06–9.42)
Black	18	7.79	8.34	(4.94–13.17)
White	100	43.29	3.18	(2.58–3.86)
Other	11	4.76	3.05	(1.53–5.47)
Unknown	78	33.77		
Total	231	100.00		
Nationality				
International	21	9.09	3.22	(2.00–4.93)
Domestic	108	46.75	2.61	(2.14–3.15)
Unknown/Unreported	102	44.16		
Total	231	100.00		
Class Standing				
Undergraduate	133	57.58	3.76	(3.15–4.45)
Graduate	39	16.88	3.13	(2.22–4.28)
Unknown/Other Unreported	59	25.54		
TOTAL	231	100.00		

*per 100,000 students.

campuses is also lower than the average U.S. population suicide rate for age groups 15-24, 25-34, 35-44, and 45-54 for males and females which was about 17/100,000 based on National Institute of Mental Health (NIMH) data from 2017 (National Institute of Mental Health, n.d.). A weighted average of the NIMH suicide rates by age group was calculated using age percentage distribution data published by the U.S. Census Bureau (Census Bureau, 2019), finding the weighted average suicide rate for age groups 15-24, 25-34, 35-44, 45-54, and 55+ was 14.72/100,000, which is still higher than 5.60/100,000.[1]

In other words, the overall average suicide rate at Big Ten college campuses was 39.4% of the U.S. population national average. Additionally, the overall average suicide rate at Big Ten college campuses is 38.0% of the weighted average U.S. population suicide rate for college-aged individuals. Taken from a different perspective, the U.S. population national average suicide rate is about 254% higher than the average suicide rate in Big Ten universities. The weighted average U.S. population suicide rate for college-aged individuals is 263% higher than the suicide rate at Big Ten universities.

The NCHS identified a 35% increase in suicide rates in 19 years from 1999 to 2018 for the U.S. population. Conversely, the suicide rate in Big Ten college campuses has decreased by 25.3% in 30 years.

Comparison of Percentages

Percentages of deaths by suicide by gender, race, nationality, and class standing were calculated (Table D-2). When comparing percentages of deaths by suicide by gender identity, the majority of deaths by suicide occurred in males (67.53%) and it is higher relative to male representation on campus (51.18%). The majority of deaths by suicide by race occurred in White students (43.29%), which is lower relative to White students' representation on campus (i.e., 74.70%). Asian students made up 10.39% of deaths by suicide on campus, making them the second largest racial group represented in deaths by suicide; this is somewhat similar to Asian students' representation on campus (8.99%).

In comparing international students with domestic students, there was a higher percentage of deaths by suicide in domestic students (46.75%). Finally, a comparison by class standing indicates that undergraduate students make up the majority of deaths by suicides in college campuses (57.58%), which is lower relative to their representation on campus (i.e., 73.95%).

---

[1] These data from the U.S. Census Bureau were obtained from the "Current Population Survey" from October 2018 (Census Bureau, 2019). Data were provided by respondents from more than 56,000 families across the United States who completed follow-up interviews providing information, among other topics, about student status of individuals in the family. These data were compared to enrollment figures across Big Ten Universities, confirming that the number of students in each age group nation-wide is consistent with the number of students in these age groups across the Big Ten universities.

Comparison of Rates

Suicide rates and Poisson 95% Confidence Intervals (CIs) for gender, race, nationality, and class standing were also calculated (Table 2) using the Epidemiology Tools package R (Aragon, 2020; R Core Team, 2020). Poisson 95% CIs that are not overlapping signify that the rates are significantly different. For gender, the suicide rates for female (1.72/100,000) and male (6.37/100,000) students are significantly different, indicating that male university students have a higher suicide rate than female students. Regarding race, the suicide rates for Asian (6.33/100,000) and Black (8.34/100,000) students are significantly different from the rates for White students (3.18/100,000), but not from each other. As such, the data indicate that while most deaths by suicide in college campuses occur in White students (i.e., 43.29%), the suicide rate of White students is significantly lower than for Asian and Black students. The suicide rates for Black and Asian students were the highest suicide rates for race.

Suicide rates for which CIs overlapped were further explored using the Exact Rate Ratio Test R package using Python[2] (Fay, 2014; PSF, 2020). The results confirmed that there were no significant differences in the suicide rates for undergraduate (3.76/100,000) and graduate students (3.13/100,000). There were also no significant differences in the suicide rates for international (3.22/100,000) and domestic students (2.61/100,000). Regarding race, the results confirmed that the suicide rate for students in the "Other" race category (3.05/100,000) was not significantly different from the suicide rate of White students and Asian students, but the suicide rate was significantly different ($p < 0.05$) from Black students.

Limitations

One of the most noteworthy limitations of the current report is the potential inaccuracy of the data reported on suicide incidents in college campuses. As expressed by Silverman at al. (1997), the accuracy and the level to which the data reported is complete can be of concern in suicide-related studies. Steps were taken to ensure that data were accurately entered into the database, such as constant communication between the counseling centers at the participating Big Ten universities and the strong commitment to the study by all institutions. Each university had its own internal system to ensure that the data contributed to the study and the database were correct and complete. Given that a standardized audit from the research team for each university was not performed, it is possible that some data are missing.

---

[2] The Exact Rate Ratio Test package was unavailable for R version 4.0.0, so a Python script for this package stored in GitHub repository was used and can be accessed through github.com/kad-ecoli/rateratio_test.

Another limitation to note is that some universities were unable to enter all their data into the database and only reported the number of incidents by year in their campuses. This resulted in some missing data for the analyses.

Additionally, a limitation of this study is its scope. The purpose and scope of this report is to update the previous suicide rate for 100,000 in college campuses in the United States. Analyses examining the gender, race, nationality, and class standing suicide rates and percentages were also performed to understand the demographic composition of Big Ten universities and of students who have died by suicide. However, this report does not seek to prove causality or draw any conclusions about motive.

Conclusion

The growing discussion of mental health in recent years has led to closer attention to the mental health issues and struggles of college students, including deaths by suicide. The current report seeks to update data on deaths by suicide in Big Ten universities. Silverman et al. (1997) published, arguably, the most comprehensive study on deaths by suicide in college campuses. Silverman et al. (1997) collected data from 12 Big Ten universities from 1980 to 1990, finding that the suicide rate in college campuses was 7.5/100,000. This was lower than the U.S. population average suicide rate at the time, which was 15/100,000 (Silverman et al., 1997). The Big Ten university counseling centers decided to continue data collection on deaths by suicide. The current study found that the updated suicide rate in college campuses using data from 2009 to 2018 was 5.6/100,000. This rate is lower than the rate reported by Silverman et al. (1997). Therefore, in about 30 years, the suicide rate in Big Ten universities has decreased 25.3%. The suicide rate found in this report is also 39.4% of the U.S. population average suicide rate in 2018, which was 14.2/100,000 (Hedegaard, Curtin, and Warner, 2020). Notably, while the suicide rates in the U.S. population increased by 35% in 19 years from 1999 to 2018 (National Institute of Mental Health, n.d), the suicide rate in Big Ten college campuses decreased by 25.3% in 30 years.

Although the goal of this report does not include an analyses of suicide ideation, motives for suicide, or general mental health in college campuses, this report highlighted important trends on deaths by suicide in college students at Big Ten universities. The updated suicide rate of 5.6/100,000 in college students and the trends on deaths by suicide identified should aide in guiding conversations about mental health trends in college campuses with more accurate information. The 25.3% decrease in the suicide rate in Big Ten universities can be evidence of the success of suicide prevention efforts taken by college campuses and counseling centers at Big Ten universities. The higher suicide rates found in this report for certain populations, such as male students and Asian and Black students, should be further explored and should be taken into consideration as universities and counseling centers continue their active efforts in suicide prevention education.

REFERENCES

Aragon, T. J. 2020. epitools: Epidemiology tools. R package version 0.5-10.1. https://cran.r-project.org/web/packages/epitools/epitools.pdf (accessed January 6, 2021).

Census Bureau. 2019. School enrollment in the United States: October 2018 – detailed tables. Suitland, MD. https://www.census.gov/data/tables/2018/demo/school-enrollment/2018-cps.html (accessed January 6, 2021).

Fay, M. 2014. rateratio.test: Exact rate ratio test. R package version 1.0-2. https://cran.r-project.org/web/packages/rateratio.test/index.html (accessed January 6, 2021).

Hedegaard, H., S. C. Curtin, and M. Warner. 2020. Increase in suicide mortality in the United States, 1999–2018. NCHS Data Brief, no. 362. Hyattsville, MD: National Center for Health Statistics. https://www.cdc.gov/nchs/products/databriefs/db362.htm (accessed January 6, 2021).

NIMH (National Institute of Mental Health). n.d. Suicide. Bethesda, MD. https://www.nimh.nih.gov/health/statistics/suicide.shtml (accessed January 6, 2021).

PSF (Python Software Foundation). 2020. Python language reference, version 3.7.6. http://www.python.org (accessed January 6, 2021).

R Core Team. 2020. R: A language and environment for statistical computing. Vienna, Austria: R Foundation for Statistical Computing. https://www.R-project.org/ (accessed January 6, 2021).

Silverman, M. M., P. M. Meyer, F. Sloane, M. Raffel, and D. M. Pratt. 1997. The Big Ten student suicide study: A 10-year study on suicides on Midwestern university campuses. *Suicide and Life Threatening Behavior* 2:285-303.